Dr. Zizmor's Brand-Name Guide to Beauty Aids

Dr. Zizmor's Brand-Name Guide to Beauty Aids

And Everything You Want to Know About Them and Whether There's Anything There That'll Hurt You and Most of All Whether They Really Do All (or Even Some) of the Things for You that the Labels Say They Do

Jonathan Zizmor, M.D., and John Foreman

HARPER & ROW, PUBLISHERS

New York, Hagerstown, San Francisco, London

Portions of this work originally appeared in *Woman's Day*.

DR. ZIZMOR'S BRAND-NAME GUIDE TO BEAUTY AIDS. Copyright © 1978 by Jonathan Zizmor, M.D., and John Foreman. All rights reserved. Printed in the United States of America. No part of this book may be used or reproduced in any manner whatsoever without written permission except in the case of brief quotations embodied in critical articles and reviews. For information address Harper & Row, Publishers, Inc., 10 East 53rd Street, New York, N.Y. 10022. Published simultaneously in Canada by Fitzhenry & Whiteside Limited, Toronto.

FIRST EDITION

Designed by Janice Stern

Library of Congress Cataloging in Publication Data

Zizmor, Jonathan.
    Dr. Zizmor's Brand-name guide to beauty aids and everything you wanted to know about them and whether there's anything there that'll hurt you and, most of all, whether they really do all (or even some) of the things for you that the labels say they do.

    Includes index.
    1. Toilet preparations. 2. Cosmetics. I. Foreman, John, 1945–   joint author. II. Title.
III. Title: Brand-name guide to beauty aids . . . RA780.Z59   613'.488   78–2170
ISBN 0-06-014802-0   78 79 80 81 82 10 9 8 7 6 5 4 3 2 1
ISBN 0-06-090655-3 Pbk   78 79 80 81 82 10 9 8 7 6 5 4 3 2 1

Contents

	INTRODUCTION: THE PURPOSE OF THIS BOOK	1
1	KEEPING FACE AND BODY CLEAN	11
2	SHAVING AND HAIR REMOVAL	29
3	PERFUMES AND COLOGNES FOR MEN AND WOMEN	41
4	DEODORANTS, ANTI-PERSPIRANTS, FEMININE HYGIENE PREPARATIONS AND DOUCHES	57
5	CREAMS AND LOTIONS	66
6	TEETH AND BREATH	83
7	MAKEUP	92
8	FINGERNAIL PRODUCTS	107
9	HAIR CARE AND COLORING PRODUCTS	115
10	ACNE PREPARATIONS	142
11	PRODUCTS FOR THE FEET	149
12	WART REMEDIES	155
13	SUN CARE PRODUCTS	159
14	MASKS	168
15	GROOMING IMPLEMENTS AND APPLIANCES	172
	INDEX	179

INTRODUCTION

The Purpose of This Book

We live today in a culture that places extraordinary emphasis on clean smells and good looks. And that's not totally unreasonable, I suppose. Surely it's preferable that one's underarms have the aroma of, say, freshly sliced limes, than that of moldy hay. And doesn't everyone want shining hair and minty breath? Who wants to look—or smell—like a pair of drying overshoes?

Well, this is a good thing—up to a point. God Himself is regularly cited as endorsing cleanliness. But things may now be going too far, and advertising copywriters and cosmetics salespeople are today treading paths that angels have always wisely avoided. The fact is the consuming public is almost wholly in the medically uneducated hands of these people. What's worse, the promoters are too often themselves true believers in their pseudoscientific pursuits. The cleverly worded claims on the sides of today's seductively packaged cosmetics and beauty aids are irresistible—even to the people who wrote them. The medical merits of most beauty aids, or their known degree of effectiveness, rarely play any part at all in the average consumer's decisionmaking process.

What's Really "Safe"?

In reaction to this situation there has evolved in recent years a body of consumers who are very consciously leery of cosmetics and beauty aids. These people are careful not to buy just anything, nor to believe just any unsupported claim. They search instead for preparations labeled "hypoallergenic," or "dermatologist tested," or "pure," or "organic." Well, this may come as an unpleasant surprise to some, but there is not much comfort to be derived from *any* of these labels.

Let's start with "hypoallergenic," my least favorite designation. The manufacturers of virtually all the lotions and potions we buy to beautify ourselves are acutely aware of the danger of what's called "sensitization." Here is a little background: in order to have an allergic reaction (of the sort that causes redness, oozing, swelling, itching, etc.), your body must first be sensitized. In order to be sensitized, there must be some initial physical contact with a substance that

INTRODUCTION

will provoke the production of "antibodies" by your bloodstream. Once you've been sensitized, it's like cocking a gun. The next time you come in contact with the sensitizing agent, bang! You get an allergic reaction. How strong the reaction is depends on the scale of the battle going on between the offending substance and your antibodies.

Sensitization is the result of what's called the "immune response" capacity of the human body. Our systems are besieged every day by substances that could literally kill us were it not for our immune-response ability. The body's white blood cells are always on the lookout for these potential troublemakers—called "haptenes"—which they easily recognize due to their unique molecular structure. What happens when a white blood cell encounters a haptene is a sort of microscopic dance, wherein the white cell rushes up to and embraces the haptene temporarily, then releases it. To the layman (and probably to the researchers who documented this as well) what next happens must seem like magic. Having embraced the haptene usually only once, the white cell suddenly has the ability to produce an antibody, which in turn will attack the haptene whenever it next appears. What's more, the white cell retains the memory of its haptene and antibody experience and actually passes this knowledge on to other white blood cells. When the knowledge is thus spread throughout the body, thereby priming the cells for any future encounter with the haptene in question, the body is said to be "sensitized."

Allergic symptoms are the result of a sensitized person's antibodies attacking haptenes. Pus, for example, is just a surfeit of sensitized white cells drawn to a battle site by the presence of haptenes. Redness and inflammation result from an unfortunate side effect that antibodies have on blood vessels. This effect is called "vasodilatation," which means an enlargement of the vessel. The vessels don't break, but they do leak. They don't leak red blood cells, but they do leak serum, which is why allergic reactions are also characterized by oozing and "edema" (medicalese for fluid collection).

Allergic reactions may seem like a needless (if miraculous) pain in the neck. But the immune response has an overwhelmingly positive side. Besides occasional perfumes and preservative chemicals, antibodies will also attack and destroy things that can really hurt you—like dangerous disease viruses and carcinogens. The whole point of prophylactic inoculation is to introduce enough (but not too many) haptenes into the system so as to inscribe on the memory of the white blood cells the ability to produce antibodies in quantity whenever needed.

To avoid the discomfort of allergic reaction, the makers of toothpaste, antiperspirants, cheek gloss, and anything and everything else that's applied to the human body go to extraordinary lengths. They do this by long, standardized series of tests on human subjects. Interestingly, this testing process is just as exhaustive for a dimestore lipstick as it is for an esoterically named and pretentiously marketed bar of pH-balanced beauty soap. And no beauty product is

INTRODUCTION

marketed unless the test incidence of sensitization is *less* than 1 in 10,000. This is standard procedure in the industry.

So if all manufacturers test their products so rigorously, why are any of them called hypoallergenic? Well, O. K., there is a tiny handful of ingredients that actually is shunned by hypoallergenic manufacturers. But even these substances—and they include things like oil of Peru (a scent), oil of bergamot (found in most luxury perfumes), as well as a few preservatives—have an incidence of allergenicity that's less than 1 in 10,000.

The point here is that, practically speaking, the measure of extra protection afforded by products bearing the label "hypoallergenic" is negligible. It doesn't make sense to buy only this type of product when the nonhypoallergenic products—even the real cheapies—are tested just as rigorously. We have a prejudice, I think, against low-class cosmetics. Whatever they look like, and whatever criticism can be justifiably leveled at the way they are marketed, the fact remains that they are really no more likely to cause an allergic reaction than their expensive "hypoallergenic" sisters.

Paying high prices for hypoallergenic products really only means that a handful of ingredients will be dependably absent. For the great majority of people, whether these things are included or omitted makes absolutely no difference. Statistically, there is no added degree of protection in hypoallergenic products. Their only value lies in the psychological impact the word has on people unaware of standard cosmetics-testing procedures.

As for the claim that a product is "dermatologist tested," I must admit (with some embarrassment, since I am a dermatologist) that in itself this is no reason to buy anything. We dermatologists find ourselves frequently solicited by cosmetics manufacturers to give such and such product a try with patients. Handsome fees are promised to the doctor for each of his patients who tries the product in question. Naturally, the dermatologists who participate in these projects would never associate themselves with anything that inflames, discolors, or irritates the skin. But that's not to say the product does any particular good, either. About the most you can deduce from a "dermatologist tested" claim is that the package contains nothing that will cause instant pain or uglification. And that's not much of a reason to buy.

As far as "pure" or "organic" products are concerned, their success is too often tied to the degree to which potential purchasers have succumbed to promotional doublethink. These two terms manage to coalesce all society's loathing of industrial pollution and ecological ruination into a foggy determination to somehow not be a further part of it all. That which is "pure" is seen as free of the chemicals that are poisoning the rivers and fouling the air. Labels that say "organic" or "natural" suggest that a product contains no nasty synthetics whose use (or preparation) will strip away the ozone layer or cause soap bubbles in the Great Lakes.

But what these claims *really* mean is that the product is either so simple as to

INTRODUCTION

have only one or two ingredients (the erroneous assumption being that "purity" always equals "effectiveness") or that the formula contains some naturally grown item (like the cucumbers in certain facial masks). "Organic" or not, you better believe that cucumber mask contains plenty of synthetic preservatives. If it didn't, it would go rancid in less than a week. Nearly all cosmetics, in fact, are fertile beds for bacteria. If it weren't for preservatives, they would have no shelf life.

Who's Protecting the Public Interest?

If you buy beauty aids—and let's face it, almost all of us do—the biggest risk you run is not that of buying something dangerous, but rather of buying something ineffective. No cosmetics manufacturer wants to be sued by someone who got a rash from his product. They're all very sensitive on this point, which is why there is so much standard testing before any preparation hits the market. All that testing is just self-defense. But, as to whether or not a product really *does* anything—as opposed to whether or not it can hurt you—well, that's another matter.

Most consumers have the subjects of safety and efficacy blurred together. What's more, they tend to credit the government with protecting the consumer from products that don't perform well on either count. If this is your perception of our government's role in the beauty-aids industry, I want to dispel it right away. Toward that end, let me ask you now which of the following four countries you think has the *weakest* laws on cosmetics labeling and ingredient claims? Italy, Great Britain, Chile, or the United States? The answer is the United States. Ironic isn't it? I think most of us would just assume that the United States has the best-developed system of controls on everything, cosmetics included.

Actually, every other civilized country has stricter rules governing both the safety and the efficacy of cosmetics. In France, for example, advertising for cosmetics cannot even use medical terms. And by medical terms, they mean words like hypoallergenic and dandruff. Sweden actually has an ombudsman whose sole function is to protect the public from misleading or ineffective beauty aids. Australia requires all poisons to be identified as such on package labels (did you know that the benzocaine contained in certain sunburn-pain ointments is actually a poison?). And Switzerland won't even allow certain cosmetic items to be marketed as such. The Swiss categorize feminine hygiene sprays, for instance, as drugs. The value of all this categorization is that it tends to protect the public as much from useless products as from those that have a potential for dangerous side effects. In America, by contrast, cosmetics exist in a unique sort of free zone, almost immune from possibly embarrassing scrutiny by government agencies.

This situation is the logical outcome of accumulated centuries of "laissez-faire" during which medicine and cosmetics have been traditionally split apart. Ever since the famed Greek physician Galen developed cold cream in the second century

INTRODUCTION

A.D., the cosmetics industry has been creeping away from medicine. In the process, it has managed to remove itself from the scrutiny to which medical preparations are subjected. Drugs, after all, are meant to diagnose and/or relieve diseases, a serious affair. Cosmetics, on the other hand, are meant to be sprayed, rubbed, poured, or sprinkled onto the body in the hopes of cleansing, beautifying, altering one's appearance, and promoting attractiveness.

The first real law governing cosmetics wasn't enacted until the seventeenth century. It happened in Italy, where, at the time, a certain beauty wash prepared with arsenic was all the rage. Arsenic gives the complexion a ruddy glow. But the Italian beauty wash was killing so many people that the government intervened and outlawed it. This began a tradition of control that has persisted in Europe to the present day. But it has never taken strong root in independence-minded America. As it happens, the Federal Food and Drug Administration (F. D. A.) concentrates on drugs to the practical exclusion of cosmetics. It devotes but 1% of its annual budget to overseeing cosmetics safety and employs a mere thirty-four chemists to evaluate all the formulas of the scores of thousands of cosmetics products on the drugstore shelves.

As for the claims made by beauty-aids manufacturers, too many people seem convinced that "they couldn't say it if it wasn't true." However, it doesn't take too close a look to discover that advertising claims, for all their seductiveness, really promise precious little. "See if you don't like our moisturizer better than your moisturizer," "Give each lash a beautiful life of its own!" "So pure, it's transparent," "42 ways to talk with your eyes," "Because the way to say 'Good night' to your skin is not the way to say 'Good morning'," "New from _____ research." These phrases were chosen at random from cosmetics ads in current magazines; more than $20 billion will be spent this year to promote cosmetics products. In the context of a slick magazine ad illustrated with photos of a gorgeous woman, one tends to forget that these lead lines promise nothing at all. Who's to say if each of your lashes is not leading a "beautiful life of its own" no matter how they all look together? So what if something's "transparent"; does that say anything about the way it works? And as far as the different ways to say good night and good morning to your skin go—well, if you believe that, you'll believe anything!

The point here is that most advertising claims are impossible to nail down. For all the high-sounding prose, they really promise nothing. There's certainly nothing in any of the aforementioned claims to give the government cause to sue. If the "new" product of such and such a company's research doesn't work, it's not because the company promised you anything different. As for the models—male and female—who adorn the ads, just remember that it took six hours to get these people looking so good, and hundreds of pictures had to be taken to insure getting the one that shows the model's bone structure in the most flattering relief. The real claim of any cosmetic or beauty aid is made by the look of the package, by the image of life the model summons up in the mind of the consumer,

INTRODUCTION

and by the attractiveness and manner of the person who makes the sale.

What this all boils down to is a single hard fact. Today's cosmetics and beauty-aids consumer is on her or his own. The products may be reasonably safe, but the question remains whether or not they *do* anything. It's a confusing area, and none of the participants—manufacturers, government agencies, retail distributors, promotional copywriters, etc.—are doing much to make it any clearer. I am *not* suggesting that anyone is intentionally throwing up a smokescreen in order to fob useless products off on an unsuspecting public. The true state of affairs is really one of general ignorance. And it is in this context—with product claims so vague as to not even promise efficacy, and government agencies mired in a longstanding tradition of laxity—that the cosmetics and beauty-aids industry is undergoing a booming proliferation not only in unit sales but in variety of available products.

Since it is impossible to judge product quality by price, or the amount of product by the size of the package, or whether or not the stuff will even work, what is the consumer to do? Give up buying cosmetics and beauty aids? Certainly not. Judiciously used, these products can make a world of difference in the way we look—and, by extension, in the way we feel. What the consumer needs now is informed advice. Which is where this book comes in.

The Potential Dangers of Beauty Aids

Despite all the exhaustive manufacturer testing, the biggest physical danger (and again—at least statistically—it's not that big a risk) is allergic reaction. The reason is that although almost every beauty aid is already hypoallergenic, there is *always* going to be someone somewhere who'll have an allergic response to something in any formula. It's a statistical inevitability.

From the manufacturers' standpoint, the name of the game, then, is to limit the number of persons who might possibly become sensitized. Besides extensive testing, this is done by periodically changing formulas. Manufacturers make slight alterations every few years to insure that regular users won't sensitize themselves to the ingredients through overuse. Interestingly, you can sensitize yourself to anything if you use enough of it.

Besides sensitization through prolonged or short-term use, there is also the problem of "cross reactivity." This is a case of an allergic reaction stemming not from one single product, but rather from a combination of products used at one time. It is possible, for example, for a deodorant soap to cross react with a cologne or a facial cosmetic or (very frequently) with simple exposure to the sun. Result: an allergic rash.

It is an ironic coincidence that as the laws regulating drugs become increasingly strict, the major drug manufacturers continue to move into the relatively unregulated cosmetics market (Lanvin and Charles of the Ritz are owned by Squibb; Maybelline is owned by Schering-Plough; and there are many other such alliances).

INTRODUCTION

Cosmetics and beauty-aids manufacturers are, however, quite willing to cooperate with customers who have bad experiences. If unusual numbers of people have trouble with any given product, it will be pulled from the shelves, and the manufacturer will report the situation promptly to the government.

Of course, with so many preparations on the market, it's hard to generalize on the subject of allergenic ingredients. But it is helpful to point out major categories, if only to give you more of an idea of the scope of substances to which you may be sensitizing yourself.

There are, first of all, preservatives. Almost everything needs preservatives whether it's touted as "organic" or not. In fact, the nearly universal necessity of preservatives is what makes the implied purity of so many "organic" products such a joke. Preservatives can be anything from exotic chemicals to plain old citric acid. Often, preservatives are antioxidents that prevent the normal oxygen exchange processes of bacteria (BHT and BHA are widely used examples). Sometimes people who have allergic problems with a given product are really reacting to the preservatives.

There are also coloring agents and fragrances to consider. Still other chemicals are often added to control a product's pH—it'll irritate the skin be it too alkaline (high pH) or too acid (low pH)—or to aid in its processing (such as the emulsifiers that effectively combine oily and watery ingredients into a pleasant texture). Then there are substances (for example, glycerin) that stabilize moisture content, without which the product would dry up in the jar.

When you come right down to it, it's a tribute to the cosmetics industry that it can successfully market so many products that can withstand months of exposure to the air and dabbling with the fingers without either drying up or going rancid. In fact, much of the cost of any beauty aid stems from the years of formulation and testing that precede the marketing of a usable product.

Aside from the dangers of allergic reaction, other less-well-understood but still possible dangers are connected with the regular use of beauty aids. The long-term influence on the human body of many substances is subtle and unclear. Traditionally, it has been assumed (both by medical people and by the public) that those things applied to the skin's surface will not be absorbed into the body. This is why nobody ever became too upset over the presence of poisons like benzocain in sunburn remedies or mercury in hand creams or suspected carcinogens in rouges, etc. However, in a 1968 test that employed radioactively tagged cosmetics preparations, it was established beyond doubt that these substances most certainly are absorbed into the system. What's more, certain areas of the body, such as the groin and face, absorb things more quickly and more thoroughly than, say, the forearm. This test shattered the myth that the skin is a barrier between the things we put on it and the bloodstream beneath it.

Does this mean that cosmetics will hurt you? Well, no, it doesn't definitely mean that. But it does mean that all the chemicals we sprinkle and spray onto ourselves are definitely being absorbed by our systems. There may well be many

INTRODUCTION

unpredictable effects from prolonged use of certain products. Many questions concerning the carcinogenic properties of certain chemicals (as well as natural substances) remain unanswered. People laugh about things like the dye Red #2 being pulled off the market. And we've all heard how many cans of diet soda a rat would have to drink before the saccharin caused tumors in his bladder. However, people have stopped laughing about the now widely feared link between hair dyes and breast cancer. And who knows what heretofore unsuspected substance lost among the many in our complicated diet and beauty habits will be the next to prove dangerous?

The Goal of the Brand-Name Guide to Beauty Aids

On July 1, 1977, a new and (in terms of the history of beauty-aids regulations in the United States) precedent-shattering law appeared on the statute books. This law requires cosmetics and beauty-aids manufacturers to list the contents of their products on the label. An excellent book titled *A Consumer's Dictionary of Cosmetic Ingredients* by Ruth Winter (Crown, 1977) explains just what every one of the ingredients you're likely to encounter really is. With this book it is possible to identify active ingredients and choose those products that give you the most action for the least money.

My own goal, however, is to read the labels for you, taking into consideration that things like the pleasant scents and elegant packages have their legitimate place in the world. With the increasing availability of disposable income, the evolution of a cosmetics market for men, the increase in the number of working women, the continued population growth, plus the heavy—and sometimes heavy-handed—promotional campaigns (six of the nation's ten top advertisers are in the cosmetics business), the consumer faces what amounts to a juggernaut. This burgeoning industry even has the remarkable ability to create markets that never before existed—witness the recent history of feminine hygiene products.

This is the reason for the book you hold in your hands. It is a guidebook in the purest sense of the word. Its real genesis was many years ago when I first began my own practice. Despite having spent what seemed like a lifetime in medical school, I found myself stumped by seemingly simple questions about the most mundane cosmetic creams and lotions. Not only did I not have the answers, nobody else seemed to, either. Books on the subject were (and still are) scarce. Those I discovered were usually painfully erudite and more concerned with how to mix the stuff up than with what the effects of its use might or might not be.

The present volume represents what I believe to be the first comprehensive popular guide to beauty aids of the sort we all buy every week. There are no axes being ground on these pages, nor is there any allegiance to organic or natural products for their own sake. My only desire is to recommend the things that work best and/or those that are particularly pleasant to use.

INTRODUCTION

Zizmor's All-Purpose Compress

Here's a tried and true compress formula that soothes allergic-type rashes on the skin. I've placed it here at the end of the Introduction for easy reference.

Take a quart container—any bottle or pitcher of approximate size will do—and fill it 95% with crushed ice. Then add about a tablespoon of salt, a teacup of skim milk, and shake or stir it up well. No great accuracy is required in measuring these ingredients.

Soak a cloth in the compress mixture and hold it onto the affected area for ten or fifteen minutes. Do this three or four times daily. The effect is wonderfully soothing—and it works equally well for sunburn and poison ivy, too.

You should, of course, permanently stop using whatever it was that caused the rash in the first place. It's also a good idea to write to the F. D. A. and/or the manufacturer to advise them of your experience.

CHAPTER 1

Keeping Face and Body Clean

Most people bathe too much, use too much soap, and stay far too long in water that's much too hot. All of this wreaks havoc with the normal moisture content of human skin and disturbs the ordinarily benign strains of bacteria resident on the skin's surface. Human bodies were not meant to be scoured and scrubbed so—especially not with the potent chemical products we've developed.

But does this mean that you should bathe as little as possible? Obviously not, as human bodies were also not meant to live in polluted air, wear tight clothing on sweltering days, or perspire from tension, worry, and aggravation. In an ideal world, we'd all go around nearly naked, never worry at all, and punctuate every other day with an ocean plunge in cleansing, naturally antibacterial sea water. Or we'd stand beneath pure rain-swollen waterfalls. Then nobody would even need soap. The way things are, however, soap is an absolute necessity.

What exactly is soap? Mostly it's fat, the same stuff the butcher trims off a steak or a pork chop. Mixed with an alkali base (anything from sodium salts to potash) this humble animal fat constitutes the basic ingredient in every soap from the cheapest to the most luxurious.

The first soaps ever produced were, interestingly, never intended for cleaning. These early concoctions, dating from the Renaissance, were designed to bleach the hair to that delicious pale auburn shade so celebrated by artists like Titian and Botticelli. The bathless culture of that time undoubtedly needed soap for cleaning considerably more than it needed auburn hair. But the hair soaps were, in fact, far too harsh and alkaline even for hair, let alone for bathing.

What about pH?

Speaking of alkalinity, I should digress for a moment and discuss "pH," surely one of chemistry's most commercially abused concepts. The pH of any substance measures its degree of acidity or alkalinity on a scale of 1 to 14. A substance that is "pH balanced" is one that registers midway between the acidic and alkaline extremes of the pH scale. Normal alkaline substances, like most of today's soaps,

KEEPING FACE AND BODY CLEAN

have a pH of 8 or 9; extremely alkaline substances like lye have a pH of 14. Similarly, normal harmless acids like lemon juice have a pH of 5 or 6, and dangerous acids—hydrochloric, for example—are pH 1.

The slightly acid (but very nearly balanced) pH of normal human skin (about 6.8) has given rise to the contention that skin naturally possesses an "acid mantle" that must be protected from alkalinity. Advertisers have seized upon this concept and used it to distort the meaning of "pH balance." Without actually saying so, they imply that any sort of alkalinity is unduly drying and damaging to the skin. This is simply not true.

All alkaline substances (like soap) are indeed drying, because they naturally strip away oil and grease that would otherwise retard evaporation of moisture. But that certainly does not mean they'll hurt you. Human skin can easily tolerate a bit of alkaline exposure without adverse effect. The production of surface skin oil is meant to purposely offset environmental drying factors, of which exposure to alkaline substances is only one. Many "pH-balanced" products use that label only as a sales gimmick. The manufacturers add just enough acid ingredients to register favorably on a piece of litmus paper. In actual use—mixed with water, in other words—their natural alkalinity reasserts itself.

A good example of this ploy is shampoo, which is a soap-based product. The gorgeous girl in the advertisement points knowingly to the litmus paper she's just dipped in the bottle. Well, litmus readings notwithstanding, once you work that pH-balanced shampoo into a lather, the lather will be decidedly alkaline, because virtually *all* soaps and shampoos are alkaline. They couldn't clean away dirt and oil if they weren't. And there's nothing dermatologically wrong with alkalinity.

There is, however, something wrong with products that are sold at inflated prices by virtue of artfully phrased but essentially meaningless claims about pH. I suppose there is also some danger if the purchasers of the so-called pH-balanced soaps and shampoos think the products won't be drying to the skin despite excessive use. Of course they will, because all soap is drying. With rare exception, all the hypoallergenic, organic, pH-balanced, pure, natural, and what-have-you soaps on the market are just as alkaline (and therefore drying) as a bar of Ivory. Ironically, even the few legitimately nonalkaline exceptions, for example, Neutrogena soap, are often equally drying.

Keeping Clean Without Drying Out

Soap is naturally drying to the skin, O. K. But it has to be in order to clean away oil and dirt. And besides, the sebaceous skin oil, produced by glands buried deep in the skin, provides the body with natural moisturization. There's a whole section on moisturizers in Chapter 5. For now, I want to point out that moisturizers work *not* by permeating parched skin with exotic "moisturizing" ingredients or rare suppleness-inducing oils. All they do is seal in plain old water. This is exactly

KEEPING CLEAN WITHOUT DRYING OUT

what sebaceous skin oil does naturally, unless your oil glands aren't producing enough of it (due, for example, to advancing age or genetic inheritance) or unless you're bathing so much, or using so much soap, or such hot water that you're depleting your own body's natural supply of moisturizer—namely sebaceous skin oil.

Long, hot baths, I regret to say, are about the worst thing you can do to your skin. They may be relaxing (as opposed to refreshing), but, ironically, they are extremely dehydrating. Look what happens to the fingertips—those "prune fingers"—after a long, hot bath. The wrinkles are caused by dehydration. Hot water opens the pores. Once you're out of that bath, the bathwater starts evaporating both off and out of your skin at a rapid rate. The hotter the bathwater, the more open the pores, and the faster the evaporation, especially if there's hardly any skin oil left to retard it.

The prescription for most dry skin is less soap, shorter baths or showers, and slightly cooler bathwater. If you have no problems at all with dry skin, then you should keep on doing exactly what you're doing right now. But if your skin is dry, the first thing to do—before spending money on moisturizers—is modify your bathing habits.

Besides being naturally drying, soap interferes somewhat with the skin's "homeostasis," or normal status quo. This it does by virtue of its mildly antibacterial nature. Whether or not it contains antibacterial additives, soap itself depletes to some degree the skin's surface bacteria count. The surface bacteria rapidly replenish themselves after soap and water washing. However, if you overuse soap you really can deplete certain benign strains of surface bacteria, which can then be replaced by less desirable strains. It's very common, in fact, for people who overbathe to suffer from rashy infectious impetigo and fungus infections in addition to excessive dryness.

The drying and antibacterial effects of soap are common knowledge. Unfortunately, too many people take these facts and draw an entirely false conclusion—that they shouldn't use soap at all. I want to refute this misconception vigorously, because soap is a necessity, which, when used moderately, won't hurt you in the least. Even on your face.

The best reason to use soap is that there is nothing else that will really get you clean. I think immediately of all the cleansing creams on the market. Many of these creams do indeed dissolve makeup efficiently, but they will not get your skin clean, nor will they unclog your pores. To get your skin really clean, there simply is no acceptable substitute for soap.

Next is the question of soap's drying effect. Well, unless you overuse soap, your own oil glands are usually quite able to promptly replenish whatever skin oil is washed away. Even sluggish oil glands are rarely a reason not to use soap; go ahead and wash and get clean, *then* use a moisturizer to seal in your bath moisture just as your own skin oil would if you had enough of it.

As for soap's antibacterial nature, let me state again that if it is used in modera-

KEEPING FACE AND BODY CLEAN

tion, it will simply not harm your skin and all the bacteria that naturally reside upon it. The bacteria will replenish themselves as a matter of course, and if you don't use too much soap, there's no reason to expect the appearance of any new or unwelcome strains.

In the eight sections that follow I've described all the soaps and bath products that you're most likely to see in magazine and television ads and on pharmacy, supermarket, and department-store shelves. Of course, products come and go. But, by the time you've finished this chapter, I think you'll be able to recognize which sorts of products work, which don't, and why. The eight sections are as follows:

(1) General-Use Soaps for Normal or Oily Skin
(2) Dry-Skin Soaps
(3) Deodorant Soaps
(4) Fragrance Soaps
(5) Beauty Grains
(6) Bathwater Additives
(7) Bathing Aids
(8) Specialty Soaps

General-Use Soaps for Normal or Oily Skin

The soaps in this category all have the virtue of simplicity, which is precisely why they appeal to my medical instincts. Nearly every other soap on the market—whether it's called "dry skin," "organic," "pH balanced," "deodorant," or what-else-have-you—is simply plain old soap with something added. The value of these added ingredients, as we'll see, is often doubtful.

The reason simple soaps are best is that the fewer the ingredients, the less chance of adverse skin reaction to any one of them. As we move through the categories that follow, you'll learn more about what some of the extra ingredients are. First, though, in this simplest category, I give my unqualified top recommendation to IVORY. This is an excellent all-around soap containing nothing unnatural or irritating—and what's more, it's very reasonably priced (dare I say cheap?) and readily available in supermarkets everywhere. Also, it floats in the tub, and it resists the sort of between-bath/shower melting that plagues so many other soap formulas. In terms of price and straightforward effectiveness on bodies, faces, and yes, even hair, I think it's one of the best values in this or any other market.

I don't reserve my praise solely for Ivory. Just as good—and just as melt resistant—is LIFEBUOY. Again, this is a product that's widely available and quite reasonably priced. Lifebuoy claims that it "keeps you smelling clean," which it does, but not by means of chemical additives. Quite simply, it works because it's a well-made, uncomplicated bar of soap and nothing else.

GENERAL-USE SOAPS FOR NORMAL OR OILY SKIN

I also give high marks to CAMAY for much the same reasons. In addition to being another low-priced standard brand, available in supermarkets everywhere, Camay also offers you the choice of blue, pink, yellow, green, and white bars. It's billed as the "soap of beautiful women," to which claim I would add the adjective "sensible." Obviously, Camay is just as good for men.

We now come to NEUTROGENA, a brand name affixed to several unusual soaps. Neutrogena has a very simple patented formula that really is nonalkaline. This soap is described as nondetergent (which means approximately the same thing as nonalkaline), nonmedicated, nonirritating, and nondrying (even though, strictly speaking, anything that strips away oil *is* drying). Neutrogena is a transparent bar whose formula originated in Belgium. Maybe that's why it's so expensive (nearly three times the cost of a bar of Ivory or Camay). I personally have high regard for Neutrogena. If you like using it and don't mind paying the surcharge, I say go right ahead. The basic model of Neutrogena is an attractively boxed bar usually sold in pharmacies. The firm also makes a dry-skin soap and a baby soap, about which more later. The Neutrogena formula, based on a chemical called ethanolamine, is unlike most soap formulas. But despite its nonalkalinity, it's still a good, gentle cleanser. Unfortunately, the bars have a tendency to get goopy in the soap dish.

These four are my top choices. But there are other soaps in the good-for-nearly-everybody category that also deserve mention. CONTI CASTILE SOAP is more expensive than Ivory, but not by much. It's an old standby—you can find it in drugstores everywhere—and the bar is free of superfluous chemical additives. Castile soaps are made from olive oil (simply a substitute for animal fat) and are named for the Spanish province where they were first developed. I'm also a big fan of AVON products. So, if the Avon lady happens by, I heartily recommend the CLEAR SKIN soap, which is mildly abrasive, mildly expensive, and comes in a melt-resistant bar with an uncluttered formula.

The prices of the soaps we've been discussing so far fall mostly within the 30¢ to $1 range, give or take a little, and they all do their job excellently. But where soap prices are concerned, the sky's the limit. High in the luxury range dwell such products as CLINIQUE MEN'S FACE SOAP and CLINIQUE SOAP EXTRA STRENGTH. Clinique is the Chivas Regal of soaps. A large bar of either, available only where Clinique products are sold (usually fancy department stores and quality pharmacies), will cost from $7 to $8! The bars are packaged in highly designed plastic containers whose outer wrappings make all sorts of claims that the product is hypoallergenic and dermatologist tested. Strictly speaking, all these claims are true. Clinique soaps work well on average and oily skins. And, although these soaps are 100% fragrance free, they even manage to smell like a million dollars. But is the extra cost justified? You'll have to come up with your own answer to that one. Just remember that Clinique neither cleans nor protects skin any better than Ivory.

KEEPING FACE AND BODY CLEAN

Dry-Skin Soaps

Several factors account for dry skin. The first is advancing age. As the years pass, a gradual and entirely normal decline in the activity of the skin's sebaceous oil glands occurs. The amount of drying that accompanies this drop in the level of skin oil varies considerably from person to person. Some see wrinkles and feel an uncomfortable tautness. Others notice hardly any change. Your own experience will largely be a function of your genetic heritage, specifically as it affects the performance of your oil glands.

The second major factor that contributes to dryness is overwashing. Many people are the cause of their own dry-skin problem for the reason mentioned several times already—namely, a fixation with cleanliness. These people aren't just clean, they've literally scoured themselves dry. Many of them probably have rather normal skin that could tolerate any general-use soap if it were used in moderation.

The third major cause of dryness is environment. This can mean living in a desert and subjecting the skin to hot sun and constantly parched air, or working in a sealed glass office tower whose ventilation system removes every drop of moisture from the air. Instead of buying nondrying soap, you might be well advised to try to modify your environment. Plants always help the moisture content of any room—the more the better. Setting out shallow tubs of water helps, too. As the water evaporates, it naturally humidifies the room. Electric room humidifiers do the same thing.

What's different about dry-skin soaps? Only one thing: They contain a little lubricating oil of some sort. Otherwise, they are essentially no different from general-use soaps. No matter what the manufacturer says, a dry-skin soap formulation will still tend to dry and dehydrate the skin. Even oil-laden soap is still soap, and soap is drying by nature. But, because of the added oil, the drying effect is retarded a bit since some of the oil will stay on the skin and discourage moisture evaporation.

If you are having trouble with dry skin, take some simple precautions. First, try to eliminate those causes of dryness that are within your power to eliminate—like overwashing, overly dehumidified air, excessive sun exposure, etc. Second, try bathing less. If you can, do it only every other day. And whenever you bathe or shower, keep it short. The longer you soak, the more pronounced the degree of afterbath dehydration. Third, keep the water a little on the cool side, since high water temperature also promotes afterbath dehydration. Fourth, use less soap. Only lather yourself once, regardless of what the label says. And fifth, use a moisturizer (recommendations in Chapter 5). After your bath or shower, you'll have about twenty minutes (at the most) to seal moisture into the stratum corneum, or upper layers of the skin. Pat (don't rub) yourself dry, and use your moisturizer to seal in water that would otherwise be lost by evaporation. This

DRY-SKIN SOAPS

procedure is as valid for hand washing as it is for baths and showers. I see many compulsive hand washers who actually think their habitual washing will moisturize their uncomfortably dry hands. Of course, just the opposite is true.

I don't feel there's any medical justification for chasing all over town for an extra-special, hypo-tested bar of dry-skin soap. Remember, there is no evidence to suggest that *any* of the different oils contained in these soaps is superior to any other as far as smoothing skin and holding in moisture goes. There's simply no reason to spend a fortune for any dry-skin soap when you can pick up a generous-size bar of TONE in the supermarket for under a dollar. Tone, manufactured by the same people who make Dial (about which more later), is my favorite dry-skin soap because of its simple formula—pure soap plus coconut oil. It's also well priced and available almost everywhere. Proper and moderate washing with this kind of soap is the simple answer to the majority of dry-skin problems.

A soap that's oilier than Tone—because it is 7½% polyunsaturated vegetable oils—is OILATUM. It does everything Tone does, and it advertises itself as lubricating and soothing to sensitive or irritated skin. I'll buy that; it's a good product.

Also in the highly recommended category is CARESS, a product of the enormous Lever Brothers Company. Caress is, once again, plain old soap, this time with the addition of mineral oil. It's a good product with an attractively low price, and it's very helpful for dry skin.

PEARS NATURAL TRANSPARENT SOAP, sold usually in pharmacies, has been manufactured in England since 1789. The manufacturer claims that it takes three months of aging and mellowing for the soap to achieve its celebrated transparence. Well, be that as it may, I personally like Pears because it contains glycerine and oil of cedar, two soothing oils. It also contains thyme, but I'm not sure just why. Pears costs about twice as much as Tone or Caress, but it's a good luxury choice. Unfortunately, it tends to melt in the soap dish.

Still in the highly recommended category are JOHNSON & JOHNSON BABY SOAP (very mild and resonably priced; available usually in pharmacies) and NEUTROGENA BABY SOAP (a little pricier, but also mild, pure, and available in pharmacies). Now that football stars are on television telling the world that they use baby shampoo, there should be no reluctance among adults in general to use baby soap on their skin.

The Neutrogena Corp. makes many specialized products, all of which are good. For example, NEUTROGENA DRY SKIN SOAP, which, like Pears, tends to melt easily. However, I like the basic formula—it's made from a hydrophilic (water-attracting) emollient (skin smoother) called ethanolamine—and the dry-skin formula contains oils not found in the Neutrogena baby bar. These oils are coconut, castor, and synthetic purcellin, as well as a bit of glycerine and tallow. Combined with a truly nonalkaline base (one of the few in existence), these make Neutrogena Dry Skin Soap very soothing to extra dry or sensitive skin. Like all Neutrogena products, it's carried in drugstores, and it's a bit expensive.

KEEPING FACE AND BODY CLEAN

The next soap is an old standby that contains lanolin. It's SHEPARD'S MOISTURIZING SOAP, whose pleasantly scented, moderately priced bars are sold in drugstores. And, of course, there's Avon's RICH MOISTURE BATH BAR, which I think is a good and effective product, as is nearly everything else that bears the Avon label.

So much for my personal favorites. If, however, you're using DOVE or JERGEN'S (both big supermarket sellers) you're getting a good buy on a good bar of soap. If you like them, there's surely no compelling reason to change. NIVEA CREME SOAP, sold in pharmacies, is also good for dry skin and is priced quite reasonably. PHYSICIAN'S & SURGEON'S SOAP, called "P & S" for short, costs almost twice as much as a bar of Nivea, but it contains soothing glycerine and no artificial chemical additives. Sold mostly in drugstores, P & S has been popular for a very long time—since 1888.

Now we begin to move into an area where the advertising claims are as insubstantial as soap bubbles. Often the soaps in question work well enough, but the outrageous claims detract from their credibility. FORMULA 405 SOAP, for example, has an impressive-sounding name and a steep price but contains nothing to make it worth three times as much as Tone or Dove. BASIS SOAP is "superfatted" and claims to protect skin from the ordinary drying effect of soap, but, of course, any soap with added oil or fat will do that. Basis seems to suggest that it will not dry the skin at all, which is simply not true. All soap is drying to some degree, even superfatted Basis.

Although I like P & S, the manufacturers of this soap also market something called OATMEAL AND BRAN SOAP. I suppose a name like this appeals to people who are convinced that oatmeal and bran are both natural and safe. Well, this happens to be true, but what it has to do with their value in a soap is quite beyond me. I don't think they do a thing, at least not for dry skin.

And, well, we could go on ad infinitum with soaps that are O. K. but not all they say they are. Why is MAZON MEDICATED SOAP good "for tender skin"? Because it has a little oil in it. Why is ESOTÉRICA SOAP "for women who need dry skin therapy"? Because it has a little oil in it too. And why does ALPHA KERI SOAP "thoroughly soothe" the skin? Because . . . you guessed it. Actually, I happen to like Alpha Keri Bath Oil, but, unless you're in love with the scent, there is no compelling reason to buy any of these soaps. At least not when you can get one at the supermarket that's just as good for a fraction of the cost.

How about glycerine soap? This product is usually lavishly packaged, sold in fancy drug or department stores, and makes a great gift. Glycerine is a thick and slow-flowing byproduct of fat decomposition. Despite its humble origins, glycerine is sweet to the taste (it's widely used in candy manufacture) and very soothing (in other words, it's oily) to dry skin. Many glycerine soaps are imported from Switzerland. TRUC, an outfit operating in the U. S. from Woodstock, Connecticut, distributes all kinds of glycerine soaps containing natural essences. Thus, you can buy glycerine soap made with apricot kernel oil, peach kernel oil, rosewater, wood strawberry oil, pure lemon oil, pure lime oil, even avocado oil. Glycerine soaps are quite gentle, and just as good for oily skin as they are for dry skin.

Ever since Phisohex disappeared from the drugstore shelves a short time back (because it contained hexachlorophine), we've had PHISODERM, instead. This is a fairly expensive liquid soap that comes in a bottle. It does contain petrolatum and lanolin, two very oily substances that are good for dry skin. But Phisoderm's label claims are classic examples of promotional puffery. Phisoderm contends that it protects the pH of the skin, that it is hypoallergenic, that it deep cleans while it moisturizes, and that its cleansing formula is good for skin of all ages. It also notes that the formula contains no perfume, which is probably the one thing it needs. Certainly, it can have no long-lasting effect on the pH of anybody's skin, no matter what their age. The claim to be hypoallergenic is not compelling, either, at least not to an informed consumer. As for cleaning and moisturizing at the same time—well, any soap with oil in it does that to some degree. Impressive as they are on a label, claims like this, while true, add up to precious little.

Now we blast off into the stratosphere, at least as far as price is concerned. In the rarefied bedrooms of Harold Robbins novels, one is likely to find ETHEREA OIL-CONTROL CLEANSING SOAP, an expensive bar containing "micro-encapsulated" emollients (specifically, mineral oil). Oil-Control Cleansing Soap comes in varying formulas for normal, oily, and dry skin, and like all Etherea products, it's fragrance free. Etherea soaps are all smoothly compounded and stylishly packaged. But, medically speaking, a bar of Tone or Caress is just as good.

This conclusion also applies to the *ne plus ultra* of dry-skin soaps, CLINIQUE SOAP MILD. This time a bar costs almost $8. It's a large bar, but. . . . Does the posh atmosphere of the department stores that carry Clinique justify this price? I don't think so. Does the hypoallergenic, 100% fragrance-free, dermatologist-tested formula warrant it? Again, I don't think so. Despite all this, some people just adore Clinique products and wouldn't dream of using any other type of soap. If they can afford it, more power to them.

As we will see in our discussion of moisturizers (in Chapter 5), it is *not possible* to restore moisture to dry skin just by using "moisturizing" oils or specially concocted dry-skin soaps. The only thing these products do is seal *existing* moisture in by applying a thin coat of oil to the skin's surface. When you take your bath or shower, you're augmenting existing moisture, and if you seal it in with an oily moisturizer, or use a soap that contains oil, you will retard the rate of afterbath dehydration.

Now, with all the dry-skin additives we've discussed, you may still wonder whether coconut oil really works better than mineral oil, or whether glycerine is actually preferable to castor oil, or lanolin, or petrolatum, or apricot-kernel oil, or what-have-you. Let me reiterate that the answer is no. For most people no single oily soap additive is clearly superior to the others. However, we humans have highly eccentric bodies, and one shouldn't generalize. It very often happens that a soap with one of these additives, let's say lanolin, may seem highly effective

KEEPING FACE AND BODY CLEAN

for one person. Yet for someone else the same product may not perform nearly as well as a soap with coconut oil. This is an established fact of the beauty-aids business. And it's one of the reasons there are so many different types of oil additives.

Deodorant Soaps

Deodorant soaps really work, and they are generally quite safe. Don't think, though, that there's anything too esoteric about these products. They are still nothing more than ordinary fat-based soap. But instead of added oil, they contain potent antibacterial chemicals called haligenated salicylanolides.

The only reason perspiration smells is because your skin's normal surface bacteria metabolize it. The byproducts of this metabolism are the sources of the unpleasant odor, *not* the perspiration itself (which, incidentally, is odorless when fresh). For most people, normal washing with normal soap is enough to control skin bacteria. However, some bodies seem to host more disagreeable strains of bacteria. If your odor problem does not respond to normal soap, only then would I recommend using the deodorant soaps whose chemical additives are potent bacteria killers.

Haligenated salicylanolides do have the potential to pose skin problems, as they can cause what are called "phototoxic" reactions. These are adverse skin reactions that occur only in the presence of light. Sometimes this means bad sunburns after hardly any exposure. Occasionally it means mystifying and long-lasting rashes and eruptions caused by exposure to fluorescent lighting, of all things. People who demonstrate the latter reaction are called "persistent light erupters." Fortunately, they are few in number. However, if you use deodorant soap and then go out in the sun, your chances of having a phototoxic reaction are excellent. This is why tropical resort hotels never stock guest rooms with this type of soap.

If you feel you need deodorant-soap protection, my top recommendation is DIAL, a soap that is both inexpensive and available in every supermarket. Dial contains triclocarban, a common antibacterial ingredient. It also contains fancy tallow and coconut oil, two oily substances that help make it soothing to dry skin.

There's a host of other deodorant soaps, all very similar, and all approximately as good as Dial. COAST is a new Procter and Gamble product in an attractively scented blue and white bar. A good enough deodorant soap, it contains triclocarban and is available in supermarkets. Unfortunately, the bar melts easily between baths. SAFEGUARD and ZEST are two more Procter and Gamble products. Aside from the color (Safeguard is pink and white; Zest is aqua) they're each practically identical to Coast, right down to containing triclocarban and being sold in supermarkets. The Colgate Palmolive Company makes a pair of deodorant soaps: IRISH SPRING, which contains triclocarban, and PALMOLIVE GOLD, which also contains triclocarban plus palm oil, olive oil, and glycerine. Both soaps are reasonably priced and widely available in supermarkets. If I had to choose between them, I'd take Palmolive Gold because of its oil content.

Fragrance Soaps

There is no objective basis on which to rate fragrance soaps. The one that's best is the one whose scent happens to please you the most. As a doctor, I feel that soap should be pure. Additives of any sort don't contribute to the purpose of soap, namely cleaning. And there's always the question of possible allergic reactions to an added scent.

Admittedly, not very many people are going to have allergic reactions to scented soap. But even the best quality extracts and essences can (and sometimes do) result in skin sensitization that wouldn't happen without them. So, I would urge you not to seek out a scented soap. But if you are already using one you like, chances are you'll be able to continue without any problems.

If you're determined to start using a scented soap, I recommend YARDLEY OLD ENGLISH LAVENDER FRAGRANCED SOAP. The bar is large, very reasonably priced (less than a dollar), and available in quality pharmacies. The manufacturer claims to have been making this soap the same way since 1770. It has a lovely lavender scent and is hard milled for between-bath melt resistance.

Most other fragrance soaps cost two or three times as much as Yardley. But scent and fancy packaging by definition make price a relatively unimportant item. Some brands, like ROGER & GALLET and PARFUMERIE, come in a whole range of assorted fragrances. It is possible to choose Parfumerie in varying fruit scents (fresh apple, fresh lemon, etc.) and Roger & Gallet in an assortment of floral fragrances. I admit that Roger & Gallet's packaging appeals to me, even though that has nothing to do with the soap inside.

If you're shopping for fragrance soap, you'll undoubtedly be browsing in quality drug and department stores. What's available in a given store depends entirely on the whim of the store's soap buyers. You're likely to see names like CREPE DE CHINE, MAJA, ULTIMA, ESTÉE LAUDER, HALSTON, REVLON, NORELL, etc. Remember that basically these are all just labels for ordinary soaps with a little perfume added. Don't be snowed by them. Manufacturers like to toss around important-sounding terminology. They'll call it hand soap, body soap, facial soap, fragranced soap for men, or any number of specific-sounding designations. But it's all just soap. This promotional terminology conveys a false impression of mutually exclusive categories of use. Actually, there's no medical reason not to use a body bar for washing the face, or a hand soap for washing the body, or a man's soap for washing a woman.

Most luxury scented soaps come in bar form—at a couple of bucks (and up) per bar. If you care particularly for a liquid soap, Ultima bottles LIQUID SKIM MILK SOAP in a 6-oz. plastic bottle. I am not convinced that the skim milk contained in this soap can do anything in particular for your skin. Supposedly, it provides protein, but just how this kind of protein can have any long-term effect on the skin escapes me. Ultima also makes a SKIM MILK ABRASIVE CLEANSER that comes in cream form in a tube. Again, if you like it, fine. But don't expect the skim milk to help clean your skin or to make it look any different after it's rinsed.

I mention skim milk because it's representative of the many natural-sounding additives that soap makers just love to promote. Skim milk sounds almost as if it could help you lose weight. A ridiculous idea, you may think, but no more ridiculous than putting skim milk (a substance with no cleaning attributes) into soap in the first place.

Beauty Grains

Particularly in the matter of cleansing the face, there seems to be an overwhelming prejudice against soap. This prejudice is groundless and the result of sheer misinformation. All day long I hear otherwise well informed and intelligent people confide that they would never dream of using soap on their faces. Why? Because soap is widely held to be too drying for facial skin, and/or to promote premature aging. This is simply not so.

Most people don't really understand the dynamics of dry skin, which is what's at the bottom of their antisoap prejudice. The key to keeping skin moist and supple is to maintain an adequate moisture level. In this case, moisture means water—nothing but water. All the oils and emollients contained in commercially prepared moisturizing products (which are discussed in detail in Chapter 5) only work to the extent that they *seal water into the skin*. The oils themselves don't moisturize; all they do is help prevent moisture already in the skin from evaporating.

Natural skin oils do the same job that commercial moisturizers do; namely, they retard the rate of water evaporation from the surface of the skin. It's true that soap strips away natural skin oils. But it's also true that skin oils very rapidly replenish themselves. Washing with soap won't hurt you. Even if your skin is dry and you don't have enough natural oil of your own, it's easy to follow a soap and water washing with the application of a moisturizer, thereby preventing excessive evaporation and attendant dryness.

Soap won't hurt skin under normal circumstances. Nor will it cause premature aging. Soap *will* get skin really clean—much cleaner than any cleanser, cream, or beauty grain. In fact, the main reason I like soap is because the alternatives usually do such a poor job of cleaning the face. And, especially if you wear makeup, you need to get your face clean.

Let's look for a moment at the sorts of things many people use in place of soap. First (and worst) is cold cream. Cold cream happens to be great for dissolving makeup. However, most cold creams also leave a pore-clogging emollient film. And while these creams are good at dissolving makeup, they aren't much good at removing dirt. A face that's been "cleaned" with cold cream alone will tend to retain an oily emollient residue. Particularly among younger women whose facial oil glands are still quite active, this residue can contribute to embarrassing acne flare-ups.

Cold cream should be used for makeup removal only, and after you've used it, you should wash your face thoroughly with soap and water. If the skin feels taut after washing with soap, then apply a moisturizer. The moisturizer should go on promptly after you rinse your face and pat it dry. A final rinse with cool water will tend to close the pores somewhat, which also helps discourage moisture evaporation.

Recently, many women with the antisoap prejudice have been converted to the use of "beauty grains." These products, also known as "cleansing grains," are not terribly effective. Theoretically, they work like Brillo, but they're about as abrasive as a Brillo made of noodles. Lots of people still love them, I suspect because of their good smells, attractive packaging, and spurious aura of being "good" for the skin.

What's in these "grains" that makes them abrasive? Answer: a collection of ineffective substances. For example, ARTISTRY II BEAUTY SCRUB CLEANSING TREATMENT contains almond meal: CLARITY BEAUTY BEADS are made from oatmeal flour; PRINCESS MARCELLA BORGHESE CLEAN SKIN SIMPLY SCRUB has walnut-shell powder and almond meal; DUBARRY CLEANSING GRAINS contain corn meal; etc. The big problem with these and all other beauty grains is that the abrasives they contain—their organic-sounding origins notwithstanding—aren't even as abrasive as a washcloth.

Curiously, most beauty-grain products are sold as being specially tailored for oily skin. What's peculiar about this is that they're actually full of oily pore cloggers. Honey, glycerine, oil of peppermint, and mineral oil—all of which are common beauty-grain ingredients—are hardly the thing to apply to oily skin. How can oil clean away oil? And they certainly can't clean away dirt. Problem oily skin is exactly the skin that needs soap and water cleaning the most.

Of course, beauty grains won't hurt you, and there's no doubt that they look, smell, and feel good. But for efficacy in cleaning the face, they're a bust. Let me reiterate that nothing cleans away dirt and emollient residues like soap. If you want abrasion, use a washcloth or a Buf Puf (a polyester sponge available in drugstores). Soap won't hurt your skin, and if you follow your face washing with the application of a moisturizer, it won't dry the skin.

Should everyone use a moisturizer after washing the face? No. And even people who do need moisturizers may well need them only on certain dry areas. It's typical for a face to have both problem dry *and* problem oily regions. Apply the moisturizer to the dry areas and leave the others alone. And if you have no problem dry areas, don't bother with a moisturizer at all.

Bathwater Additives

Bath oils—as well as bath beads, bath powders, and bath gels—are supposed to do two things: scent the bathwater and moisturize the skin. They do the first much better than the second.

KEEPING FACE AND BODY CLEAN

The typical bath oil (or bead or gel) is a simple compound of three main ingredients. The first is oil (either vegetable or mineral); the second is perfume (usually about 10% of volume); and the third is an emulsifier (to mix the oil and perfume and make them stick to the skin). Once they're mixed with water, oils, beads, gels, and powders are all equally effective.

Like scented soap, the advantage of commercially prepared bath oil is zero. You can easily make your own out of any oil in the kitchen cabinet (corn oil, safflower oil, etc.) plus a few drops of your favorite perfume or cologne. Any oil in the tub, homemade or otherwise, will indeed make your skin feel smoother after your bath. But does this mean that the skin is being efficiently moisturized? No, it does not. A greater degree of skin hydration will occur if you bathe first in plain water and then apply a moisturizer afterward. Besides, for some women, frequent bathing with bath oils causes vaginitis.

The ideal way to use bath oil for moisturization is to bathe first, then get out of the tub and rub oil on the skin. But it's silly to do that with so many good moisturizers available. So, if you are going to use bath oils, in most cases you'll be doing so for the scent; you can use about half the amount the directions tell you to and still get the desired smell. Also, people tend to tire easily of bath oils. Therefore, don't buy big sizes, even if they seem to be a bargain.

The same advice applies to bath salts. Since many of these products contain no oil at all, they are not good moisturizers by definition, but even those that contain oil don't do the job as efficiently as an afterbath moisturizer. Bath salts usually come in powdered form, and, in my opinion, their value lies chiefly in the pleasure you may derive from their scent. The major ingredients in bath salts are rock salt, perfume, sodium bicarbonate (for those that effervesce in the tub), and, sometimes, various mineral salts. Pleasant? yes; moisturizing? not very.

Now for my favorites:

CALGON BOUQUET BATH appeals to me because it has a pleasant flowery scent and a low price. It comes in powder form, and, like other Calgon products, it's widely available in drugstores. If the Bouquet Bath doesn't suit you, Calgon also makes CITRUS, FLORAL, and PEACH bubble baths. They're all inexpensive, and they all claim to pamper the body and soothe the soul at the same time—which, if it works for you, is a bargain for under two bucks. Just as good, and just as cheap, are CALGON BATH OIL BEADS, which are slightly different in scent, but are otherwise similar to the Bouquet and bubble baths.

ALPHA KERI BATH OIL is a soothing old standby that comes in plastic bottles for the bath and handy sprays for the shower. Its green liquid contains lanolin and mineral oil, and as such it's very soothing to dry skin. Some people love the scent; others can take it or leave it. It's carried in drugstores and has a moderate price tag.

The next recommendation contains oatmeal, the sort of additive that usually makes me laugh. But the fact is that AVEENO COLLOIDAL OATMEAL is an extremely soothing bath powder. A drugstore product, this stuff is great for skin irritations

BATHWATER ADDITIVES

like sunburn or poison ivy, as well as for ordinary dryness. It does tend to make the tub extra slippery, though, so be careful.

AVON markets quite a few good, uncomplicated, reasonably priced bath oils and beads. The Avon lady is well aware that scent and image are the name of the game in bathwater additives. Thus, Avon offers products with names like Timeless, Unspoken, Sweet Honesty, Occur, and so on. They're all just fine.

Now we move into the luxury range. And what better place to start than with VITABATH GELÉE. Packaged in a variety of sizes, in both tubes and bottles, Vitabath is a European import that's been popular across the Atlantic (under the name BADEDAS) for many years. It contains lanolin, sunflower oil, and horse-chestnut extract, among other things. Maybe it's the horse chestnuts that make it smell so sensationally good. Vitabath is intended to be used in lieu of soap. And I suspect that people who use Vitabath regularly instead of soap probably weren't very dirty in the first place. The product is expensive, sold in pharmacies, and very attractive to the eye and the touch.

NEUTROGENA RAINBATH DRY SKIN BATH GEL is also intended as a soap substitute—for skin that's either too dry or irritation prone for normal bathing. I don't think many people really fall into this category, but whether you do or not, this is a pleasant bath oil for soaking or showering (in which case you apply it directly to the washcloth), and you can usually buy it in good drugstores.

So much for my favorites. I hasten now to add that my favorites are not much different from most of the other bathwater products on the drugstore shelves. Other good and reasonably priced bath beads include JERGEN BUBBLING BATH BEADS (from the same "lotion mild" people who make the famous hand cream), VASELINE BRAND INTENSIVE CARE (whose Mineral Bath Powder, Bath Beads, and Herbal Bath Beads are all good smelling and very reasonably priced), SOFTIQUE CITRUS BOUQUET BATH OIL BEADS (there's also a Softique Herbal Seas), and BATHERAPY (whose beads purport to contain minerals found in America's hot-spring spas). Similarly good products in oil form include SARDO BATH OIL CONCENTRATE (with mineral oil), TENDER TOUCH BATH OIL, FORMULA 405 BATH OIL, SYNTEX BATH OIL, and COURTESY BUBBLING BATH OIL (with coconut oil). None of these products is special, but they're all equally good.

Having already stated that scent is the name of this game, I still find myself hesitating to endorse very expensive products no matter how good they smell. But, that's my problem. If you like the scent of HALSTON MILK BATH POWDER or LANVIN MODERN BATH SALTS or TRUC FOAMING BATH GEL or ULTIMA SKIM MILK BATH OIL or NORELL PERFUMED MILK BATH, to cite only a few of the many luxuriously priced bathwater products available, then use them. But don't expect them to do anything in particular for your skin. If the perfume pleases you and you have the money, go ahead.

The promotional copy on the packaging of luxury bathwater additives seems designed to convince consumers that miracles are about to happen: "Highest quality of Swiss craftsmanship," "natural cereal derivative for soothing and cleansing," "cleanses naturally due to its unique absorptive action," "protection therapy," "locks in restored moisture balance," "freshens and silkens the skin," "contains no soaps or synthetic detergents," "for sensitive skin," etc. Don't let phrases like these confuse you. Any bath oil, bead, gel, or powder can at best do no more than temporarily add a little smoothing oil to the surface of your skin. Usually all it does is make the bathroom smell good.

Bathing Aids

This category contains products designed to rub against the skin. They demonstrate the concept of "epiabrasion," a dermatological term referring to the therapeutic effects of abrading or scrubbing the epidermis, or top layers of the skin.

The idea behind epiabrasion is scraping off surface skin cells. Dermatologically, this is absolutely sound. It accomplishes several things: (1) it encourages maintenance of a healthy cell-turnover rate (skin grows from the inside out and, as such, it constantly sheds cells from the surface); (2) it discourages acne, by removing excess oil before it has a chance to clog your pores; and (3) it stimulates the circulation and gives the skin an attractive ruddiness. Epiabrasion is as good for older people as it is for acne-prone youngsters. It helps scrape away skin lesions connected with age (like accumulated sun damage, keratoses, and liver spots) while stimulating the blood supply and encouraging the growth of healthy new skin. It also plumps up the skin cells, thereby minimizing lines and wrinkles.

Epiabrasion makes people of all ages look healthier, and I recommend it highly. But there is, of course, a danger of overdoing it. Epiabrading too much can make the skin raw and sensitive and cause a temporary burning sensation. Lessening the amount of daily rubbing—or going a few days without it—is the normal prescription. There are some people, however, whose sensitive skin just won't tolerate any epiabrasion without becoming uncomfortably irritated. This isn't abnormal; these people just shouldn't try.

People usually epiabrade only areas of problem acne or sun exposure. There is, in fact, no reason not to epiabrade the whole body, but this is unnecessary and not very convenient. Those skin areas that you do epiabrade should be rubbed vigorously—and, again, be careful not to rub yourself raw—for about a minute each morning. Depending on your skin's tolerance, you can maintain your minute scrub, or extend it up to about three minutes. Be sure the soap you use is compatible with your skin's level of oiliness.

My own favorite epiabrasion product is the BUF PUF. This nonmedicated polyester cleansing sponge has a nice uniform texture, is long lasting, and is available in drugstores for under two dollars. My second choice for price and uniformity of texture is the FULLER COMPLEXION BRUSH, but it's not easy to obtain. Only a Fuller Brush man can get it for you.

For those with a prejudice against polyester or synthetic complexion brushes, I recommend a LOOFAH. This natural fiber product (generally made by cleaning and drying the contents of certain gourds) is packaged by a variety of firms in many sizes. Like the Buf Puf, it's a drugstore item. SPA GENUINE LOOFAH, LOOFAH NATURAL BATH SPONGE, LOOFAH STRAP (which is made of rope), and LOOFAH MITT are typical products. They will, as the packages claim, improve circulation and soothe tired muscles. They will not give the body greater vigor or have any impact on "cellulite," the fortunately defunct pseudoscientific name for fat.

Loofahs and Buf Pufs are scratchy; be prepared. Natural sponges, however, are quite soft. They're also quite luxurious, fairly expensive, and available only in good department stores and fancy pharmacies. MERMAID OCEAN SPONGE, NATURAL SPONGE, or any other natural sponge is equally good. Real sponges are wonderful fun in the tub, but they do have a tendency to tear. For the purposes of epiabrasion, an ordinary washcloth is cheaper, stronger, and less scratchy than a loofah.

Finally we come to bath brushes. These are mostly for scrubbing the back, and unless you were raised with one, you probably won't miss it. Most brushes, like the MASSAGE-BRUSH, and the DRÜCKEN brush, are imported from Europe. They have synthetic bristles, cost between $5 and $10, and are available at quality drug and department stores. The Drücken brush also lets you adjust the amount of bristle exposed and thereby control hardness. Natural-bristle bath brushes are available in the same price range. I don't think there's any inherent advantage to natural bristles, although they are certainly as good as the synthetic ones.

Specialty Soaps

The half-dozen recommendations that follow really are unique, in that each fulfills a purpose that plain soap alone cannot.

LOWILA is a soapless soap formulated for highly allergic people with skin that can't tolerate normal soap. Its cleaning formula is based on mineral oil and boric acid, which act as acceptable substitutes for typical animal-fat soap ingredients. Lowila comes in a bar that must be kept dry between uses or it turns into a puddle. This soap is available in drugstores and is recommended for use *only* on extremely allergy-prone or irritated skin.

LAVA is for skin that is not particularly sensitive but is very dirty. It's a supermarket item, very abrasive, very inexpensive, and has a nice scent. Lava is my choice for heavy cleaning.

SALICYLIC ACID SOAP softens rough skin. It is excellent for use on calluses, roughened areas, acne-prone areas (since it's a good degreaser), and/or any other part of the body. There is no medical reason not to use Salicylic Acid Soap as your regular daily soap. However, people generally use it only on roughened areas until the roughened condition is overcome. Buy it at drugstores.

POLYTAR SOAP is a drugstore item made from a combination of vegetable and mineral tars. It's specially formulated for skin suffering from eczema, psoriasis, and/or seborrhea (a. k. a. dandruff). These are all basically dry-skin problems, which often respond well to the tars in this soap.

KEEPING FACE AND BODY CLEAN

SALICYLIC ACID AND SULFUR SOAP is an antiseptic OTC (over-the-counter) soap that kills funguses. It's designed primarily for home treatment of a common condition called tinea versicolor. The fungus that causes this condition is benign, but as part of its normal metabolic processes, it produces a chemical sunscreen. The result is a blotchy tan whenever the skin is exposed to the sun. Because this soap is the kind of product never advertised on television, some people think it must be a prescription item requiring a doctor's instructions for use. But it's just an old standby home cure available in almost any drugstore.

DESENEX is a name closely associated with feet (see Chapter 11: Products for the Feet), but they also make an antibacterial, antifungal bar soap. This soap has the same salutary effect on tinea versicolor as Salicylic Acid and Sulfur Soap. It can be used on the entire body (on a daily basis if desired) and is also effective against problem body odor. Both these soaps are helpful in combating athlete's foot, but there are better remedies for that ahead in Chapter 11. Desenex soap, by the way, is also a drugstore item.

CHAPTER 2

Shaving and Hair Removal

Hair can indeed be lovely. But it's a pity so much of it grows in the wrong places. This chapter surveys and evaluates the many types of products designed to render your skin smooth and unstubbled. We'll start with Preshave Preparations then move along to Razors, Razor Blades, Shaving Creams, Shaving Powders, Styptic Pencils, Aftershave Lotions, Depilatories and Epilators, and, finally, Electric Razors. The information will be equally useful to both men and women, because, marketing campaigns notwithstanding, shaving and hair removal are strictly unisex affairs.

Preshave Preparations

The lotions and powders in this category are meant for use exclusively with electric razors. They perform a necessary setting-up and astringent function and are meant to play the role that shaving cream does in wet shaving.

In order for electric razors to give a close shave on faces, underarms, legs, or anywhere else, the skin must be relatively free of oil. Only then can the hair stand up fully and present itself to the razor for a clean, low cut. Lotion preshaves are little more than alcohol-based astringents. They usually contain ingredients like menthol and camphor as well as a little scent of some kind. These added ingredients do nothing to degrease the skin or properly set up the hair, but they do make the products smell good and feel cooling. Plain alcohol would do the setting-up job just as well, but it's not as pleasant to use.

In addition to preshave lotions there are preshave powders. Unlike lotions, these products absorb skin oils instead of stripping them away. They're made primarily from talcum powder with a little added scent. Talcum powder, since it is very soothing, makes an excellent aftershave. And, in fact, the directions to most preshave talcs advise you to use them both before and after you shave.

People who own electric razors are well advised to use some kind of preshave preparation. To do so will insure a much cleaner and closer shave. Preshave products are all very simple, very similar, and not very expensive. The one that's best is the one you find most pleasant to use.

SHAVING AND HAIR REMOVAL

The J. B. Williams Co. of Cranford, New Jersey, makes a dependable and reasonably priced lotion that I recommend highly. Called WILLIAMS 'LECTRIC SHAVE, it has a simple alcohol base and does the job well. Williams also makes a FROST LIME variation of 'Lectric Shave, but I would avoid on principle products that contain lime scent. This substance can be a potent photosensitizer, which means it can precipitate a bad skin reaction in the presence of sunshine. And, anyway, the scent of the regular product is pleasant enough without the lime.

If your skin is particularly tender or prone to nicks and/or razor burn, I recommend WILLIAMS 'LECTRIC SHAVE TENDER FACE SPECIAL FORMULA. The only thing special about this formula is the addition of silicone, which noticeably improves razor glide. Although Williams directs its advertising at the male market, women who use electric razors should definitely try it.

Also good are MENNEN SKIN BRACER PRE-ELECTRIC SHAVE LOTION, OLD SPICE PRE-ELECTRIC SHAVE LOTION, and BRUT 33 PRE-ELECTRIC SHAVE. These are all inexpensive—even Brut, surprisingly enough—and they all have simple alcohol-based formulas. Old Spice, Brut, and Williams also contain isopropyl myristate, a sort of oily-type alcohol. It simultaneously degreases and promotes razor glide.

Shaving talcs, on the other hand, do much less degreasing. Since alcohol is very drying, the talcs are good for older people, whose skin is naturally dry, or for those who simply don't want to aggravate a non-age-related dry-skin problem. Among the talcs, my favorite is MENNEN SHAVE TALC, an old standby that contains a neutral coloring to hide nicks and blemishes. The cost is less than a dollar for a 4-oz. plastic dispenser, and, like all these products, it's carried in pharmacies. Also good is OLD SPICE SHAVE TALC, which has a pleasant scent but a slightly higher price.

Razors

I am concentrating here on nonelectric razors, which I prefer to electric models (details on which are at the end of this chapter) because they give a closer shave.

I feel that the best razor for men or women is the HOFFRITZ ANGLE RAZOR. It takes a standard double-edged blade but holds it in a uniquely angled mount. It's an expensive item—$20 if the case is nickel-plated brass; $13.50 if it's plastic—but it will last for a lifetime. Hoffritz makes all manner of quality utensils and sells them in Hoffritz stores around the country. This razor gets my unqualified endorsement because of its good quality and durability and the close shaves made possible by the way the angled blade fits the contours of the face.

If Hoffritz is the Cadillac of razors, then the GILLETTE SUPERADJUSTABLE is the good old Ford. This is a workhorse that's hard to beat. For a couple of dollars (for which you'll also receive a pair of Platinum Plus double-edged blades) you'll get a razor that, like the Hoffritz, will last you for the rest of your life.

Single-edge injector razors, like the SCHICK INJECTOR, are inexpensive (under two dollars) and perform adequately. They seem light to me, though, and I can't see them lasting many years. However, that's not important to everybody.

Other good razors include the WILKINSON BONDED SYSTEM (a fancy name for a razor and three blades costing around two dollars); the GILLETTE TECHMATIC (which shaves with an adjustable cutting band); and—if you don't mind the waste—any of the many disposable razors. The BIC SHAVER is a typical disposable. It costs a quarter and is good for at least two or three shaves ("Holds its edge for shave after shave," as the manufacturer puts it).

Although razors are a unisex item, I do like the FLICKER, which advertises itself as a ladies' safety shaver from the American Safety Razor Co. The design includes a useful skin shield that helps avoid nicks on underarms and legs. It's a good buy for under two dollars.

Scraping any razor across the skin is abrasive; many people wonder if it's not too abrasive. The answer, at least under normal circumstances, is no. Skin is constantly shedding dead cells from the surface. The additional abrasion of a single razor blade won't hurt you. Nor, incidentally, is there any evidence that shaving with a blade will do any of the following: (1) cause hair to grow back more rapidly; (2) enlarge pores (which are the surface openings of sweat ducts); (3) enlarge hair follicles; or (4) make hair grow back darker. The rate and quality of hair growth has nothing to do with shaving. Rather, it's a function of hair-follicle metabolism, a process regulated by hormones and nutrients in the bloodstream. These substances feed the hair follicle, which is buried deep in the lower layers of the skin, far from any contact with a razor blade. You might nick yourself with a razor blade, but usually that's your only risk.

What I *don't* like on the subject of razors is the whole "twin blade" concept. From a dermatological standpoint, dragging *two* blades across the skin is excessively abrasive. I find the incidence of razor burn and skin rash is substantially higher among those who use twin-blade razors. I actively discourage their use. You certainly don't need them to get a good shave.

It seems, though, as if everybody has jumped on the twin-blade bandwagon in the last few years. Thus many of the manufacturers of recommended regular razors also make nonrecommended twin-blade varieties. These include the GILLETTE TRAC II series, as well as the GILLETTE DISPOSABLE TWIN BLADE RAZOR and the DAISY TWIN BLADE SHAVER. Just as bad to my mind are the SCHICK SUPER II (and the LADY SCHICK SUPER II), the PERSONNA DOUBLE II (and the PERSONNA LADY, which uses twin blades), and all other types of twin-blade systems.

Razor Blades

Blade coatings really work, especially platinum and Teflon. They give a closer shave because they keep the cutting edge sharper longer. However, blade performance declines sharply after the second or third shave. Advertising claims to the contrary should be taken with large grains of salt.

The following blades are the best: GILLETTE PLATINUM PLUS BLADES; GILLETTE PLATINUM

SHAVING AND HAIR REMOVAL

PLUS INJECTOR BLADES; SCHICK SUPERCHROMIUM WITH TEFLON COATING; SCHICK PLUS PLATINUM BLADES; SCHICK PLUS PLATINUM TEFLON COATED BLADES; plus any other blade with a platinum and/or Teflon coating. These blades generally cost in the vicinity of a quarter apiece, give or take a few cents.

A wide variety of other coatings can be found on razor blades. They generally work well, even though my personal preference is for Teflon or platinum. Among the still-pretty-good alternatives are: SCHICK SUPERCHROMIUM BLADES; WILKINSON SWORDMASTER CHROMIUM BLADES; and PERSONNA 74 TUNGSTEN PLUS for regular and injector razors, to name only a few. The prices of these alternate coatings are often slightly lower than platinum or Teflon.

Uncoated blades obviously work, but the quality and closeness of even the first shave are not going to be as good as with a coated blade. There is, however, quite a cost savings with the uncoated models. WILKINSON BLADES, GILLETTE BLUE BLADES, and GILLETTE SUPER BLUE BLADES usually cost less than 15¢ per blade. GILLETTE SUPER STAINLESS BLADES and WILKINSON BONDED BLADES cost only a few pennies more, but for that money I'd go for a coated model.

Again, I think that twin parallel blades are bad for your skin and therefore advise you to steer clear of GILLETTE TWINJECTOR BLADES, GILLETTE TRAC II BLADES, SCHICK SUPER II BLADES, WILKINSON II BLADES, PERSONNA DOUBLE II BLADES, and any other twin blade, as well as the razors they fit.

Shaving Creams

The purpose of shaving cream is to give the blade a glide and make the cut smooth and easy. Hairs softened with moist shaving cream do cut more easily, but shaving cream does not remove all potential for irritation.

In fact, shaving irritation is a common sight to any dermatologist. Sometimes this means no more than an uncomfortable rash, a burning sensation, or a painful degree of sensitivity to touch. Other times, hairs can become ingrown and cause granulomas, brownish papules that are your skin's response to intrusion by a foreign object (in this case, your own hair). Especially on black skin, granulomas can often develop into unsightly wide keloidal scars.

One of the main problems to overcome in shaving is its inherent abrasiveness. Toward this end, always shave after a hot bath or shower. Hair equilibrates with its environment, which means it soaks up moisture easily, especially from a hot bath. And it's much easier to cut when swollen with moisture. If you can't bathe before shaving, then at least wash your face or legs or underarms (or whatever) with hot water and soap, or wrap the area with a towel soaked in hot tap water.

Shaving with the grain minimizes abrasion and irritation. It's not always easy to do, but try to if you can. Since skin is made raw to varying degrees by shaving, the fewer ingredients in the shaving cream the better. Menthols, citric essences, perfumes, and so forth are more a source of irritation than of comfort. As with soap, the less extra ingredients the better.

SHAVING CREAMS

Statistically, nonaerosol shave creams are less irritating than the ones in aerosol cans. Why this is true is not entirely clear. Some doctors hypothesize that the aerosol propellants can irritate skin that's been freshly scraped with a razor. Most people, however, can use aerosol shave creams without difficulty, which is fortunate, since they're so convenient.

Keeping in mind the goal of minimizing irritation wherever possible, I choose NOXZEMA MEDICATED LATHER SHAVE CREAM as my number-one choice. Don't confuse it with the aerosol Noxzema, or with the blue jar of regular Noxzema cream, either. The shave cream comes in a tube. You squeeze it onto the hand, apply to the skin with the fingers, and use a wet shaving brush to work up a lather. Noxzema's "medication" boils down to very small amounts of camphor, menthol, and various oils (eucalyptus, peppermint, clove), which account for the pleasant scent more than for any particular medicating function.

Noxzema also makes a BRUSHLESS SHAVE CREAM, which is designed to be worked into the beard (or onto the legs, etc.) with the fingers. In fact, nearly all nonaerosol shaving creams come in lather and brushless forms, each of which is equally good.

Besides Noxzema, I highly recommend the following (with their specific glide-inducing ingredients in parenthesis): GILLETTE LATHER SHAVE CREAM (with glycerine) and BRUSHLESS SHAVE CREAM (with peanut oil); PALMOLIVE LATHER SHAVE CREAM (with glycerine) and BRUSHLESS SHAVE CREAM (with mineral and olive oils); MENNEN LATHER SHAVE (with glycerine and coconut oil) and BRUSHLESS SHAVE (with glycerine and mineral oil); WILLIAMS GOLDEN YELLOW LATHER SHAVING CREAM (with glycerine, coconut oil, mineral oil, and lanolin); and BARBASOL BRUSHLESS SHAVE CREAM (with mineral oil, paraffin, cornstarch, lanolin, and talc).

Shaving soaps are just as good as creams. My top recommendations are: WILLIAMS MUG SHAVING SOAP (with tallow and coconut oil); COLGATE CUP SOAP FOR SHAVING (which is simply plain soap); and OLD SPICE SHAVING MUG SOAP (which is essentially just scented soap). All these items are to be found in drugstores, and they're *cheap*—in the best sense of the word.

Surveying a category like shaving cream makes one appreciate the dazzling degree of choice consumers have in a country like the United States. My preference on principle for non-aerosol creams notwithstanding, the aerosol models are very convenient. Most of them even have eliminated their ozone-depleting fluorocarbon propellants. Assuming that you won't have an allergic reaction to the propellants—and it's a good bet you won't—I give a strong endorsement to certain aerosols in the *regular* formula. Again, beware of lime- and lemon-scented creams; these very often cause phototoxic skin reactions—specifically rashes and shockingly bad sunburns—in combination with sunshine. As far as exotic scents go, well, chances are they won't hurt you. Still, I'd skip them on the grounds that it is always preferable to avoid putting extra chemicals on the body.

The following regular-formula aerosol shaving creams are recommended: NOXZEMA SHAVE; NOXZEMA MEDICATED SHAVE; RISE; RISE HEAVY; RISE BABY FACE (which contains light mineral oil and is, ironically, good for older people with dry skin);

SHAVING AND HAIR REMOVAL

EDGE LATHERING GEL; AQUA VELVA SILICONE LATHER SHAVE (silicone is a slippery substance that encourages razor glide); OLD SPICE (with mineral oil); GILLETTE FOAMY (with glycerine); MENNEN SOF' STROKE REGULAR SHAVE (with lanomen, a derivative of lanolin); RAPID SHAVE (with glycerine); RAPID SHAVE COLOGNE SCENT (with glycerine plus a little cologne); BARBASOL CONCENTRATED LATHER SHAVING CREAM (which contains glycerine and calls itself the "beard buster"); COLGATE INSTANT SHAVE (with coconut oil); AEROSOL REFILLS FOR SCHICK HOT LATHER DISPENSER (with glycerine, lanolin, and mineral oil); BRUT 33 CREME SHAVE; ENGLISH LEATHER POWER FOAM SHAVE CREAM (with mineral oil and glycerine); and REXALL REDI-SHAVE CREAM.

Soap, which is contained in every one of these shaving products, is really enough to produce adequate razor glide. Whether or not you need the extra glide that slippery additives like lanolin, coconut oil, silicone, or glycerine can provide is a matter of personal preference. Incidentally, I don't think any of these glide-inducing additives is inherently superior to the others.

All the aerosols recommended above are reasonable priced, which means a big can (11 ozs. or so) costs around $1.50 or less. Barbasol, Colgate, and Rexall are particularly good bargains, with the same big can costing well under a dollar.

The following shaving creams are *not* recommended: First and foremost is *The Hot One,* a weird chemical compound from Gillette. This product produces the impression of heat not by getting hot, but by making the skin burn slightly. Lots of allergic reactions have been traced to this one, and the "hot" gimmick does little or nothing to improve shaving. GILLETTE TRAC II SHAVE CREAM, with peanut and mineral oil, is not a bad product, but I dispute the validity of the whole twin-blade shaving concept. There's nothing special about this cream; one's patronage of it only perpetuates "Trac II" nonsense. ARAMIS 900 ABSOLUTE COMFORT SHAVE FOAM calls itself the "perfectly painless shave" by virtue of the benzocaine contained in its formula. Besides being a mild topical anesthetic, benzocaine is a well-known allergen. I don't know that I'd want to rub this substance on myself every day, despite the lack of any studies that prove it's dangerous to do so. What's more, the stuff is very costly. Which brings us to KANON RICH SHAVE FOAM, typical of any number of pleasant-smelling and extremely expensive shave creams. Is it worth paying ten times the price of Barbasol, or seven times the price of Rise, for this or any shaving cream? Not for me, it isn't. Especially when the difference between them is negligible.

Shaving Powder

Shaving powder is for black men worried about razor bumps. The active ingredient is thioglycolate, the same chemical found in cream hair-removal formulas (like Nair) that women use on their legs.

Razor bumps result from extra curly hair that grows back into the skin. This is particularly liable to happen after the hair is freshly shaved. The sharp edge of the cut hair can curl down onto and pierce the skin that surrounds it. As the hair grows, it burrows into the flesh and causes a razor bump. The next day's shave can turn the bump into a cut. Sometimes the body itself will react to the ingrown hair by causing what's called "folliculitis." These unsightly bumps can become inflamed and enlarged. At their worst, they can result in ugly keloidal scars.

Some black men are so prone to razor bumps that they cannot shave with a blade. That's where shaving powder comes in. Mixed with water and applied with a rubber spatula, it chemically attacks the hair without harming the skin. After two to five minutes, the edge of the spatula is used to remove the paste together with the hair.

The Carson Product Co. of Savannah, Georgia, makes a premier product, called MAGIC SHAVING POWDER. It's reasonably priced and contains, besides thioglycolate, soothing cornstarch and a fragrance. Despite the fragrance, shaving powder smells fairly bad. Magic comes in a blue can for regular beards, in a red can for extra tough beards, and in a gold can for those who like extra fragrance. Although thioglycolate won't hurt the skin, it does tenderize it somewhat. You won't be able to use normally alcoholic cologne or aftershave—which is why Magic makes their own After Shave Cream and After Shave Skin Conditioner, described below under Aftershaves.

Styptic Pencils

Touching the point of a styptic pencil to a shaving cut will stop the bleeding immediately. It costs little more than a quarter, is available in drugstores, and lasts nearly a lifetime, so a styptic pencil is a must for anyone who repeatedly cuts or nicks himself or herself with a razor. The active ingredient is usually aluminum sulphate, but any salt of aluminum does the job equally well. Lewer Drug Products of New York City makes a "NEW AND IMPROVED" STYPTIC PENCIL. (I don't think there is such a thing as a bad one.)

Aftershaves

What does an aftershave really do? Let's look at the labels and see what they say. "Leaves face feeling fit and fresh," "strengthens and tones your skin," "brisk when applied, it mellows into a sophisticated subtleness," "gives you the freshness of the open sea," "wakes you up like a slap in the face." If you can draw any conclusions from these claims, more power to you.

Aftershaves are nothing more than perfume and alcohol, with occasional dashes of things like propylene glycol or lanolin or glycerine (for soothing, which they don't do well) or menthol (for a cooling sensation). Aftershaves contain more pure fragrance than cologne, and less pure fragrance than perfume. Mostly, they are alcoholic astringents that tone the skin by temporarily tightening the pores. And, of course, they smell good.

SHAVING AND HAIR REMOVAL

It is curious indeed that so many of them claim to be soothing. I can't imagine alcohol being anything but burning when applied to skin that's just had a razor dragged across it. Before public consciousness was media-blitzed into believing in aftershaves, people used water or talcum powder, both considerably more sensible than alcohol if one's desire is to soothe raw skin. Aftershaves have survived and flourished purely on the strength of their pleasant smell. Frankly, I think you're better off using cologne, which smells just as good and usually costs less per ounce.

Although aftershave lotions are not necessary, I recommend several good, cheap ones that amount to low-cost cologne. My favorite is LILAC VEGETAL, a French import found in better drugstores that's also cheap (12 ozs. for a little more than two dollars) and very pleasant smelling. It's nothing but alcohol and lilac fragrance. After that, I'd pick AQUA VELVA in either the ICE BLUE or the newer REDWOOD fragrance. Aqua Velva has a little glycerine (for soothing) and menthol (for a bit of a kick), two ingredients that would actually seem to work at cross purposes. Still, the price is low, the availability nearly universal (in drugstores), and the smell quite pleasant. I also recommend ST. THOMAS VIRGIN ISLAND GENUINE IMPORTED BAY RUM. Of course there's no rum in it, but the smell is tropically handsome, the price is exceptionally low (about two dollars for 16 ozs.), and the availability (again in drugstores) quite good.

Let me make special note of MAGIC AFTERSHAVE SKIN CONDITIONER and MAGIC COOLING SOOTHING AFTER SHAVE CREAM. These are nonalcoholic compounds—both contain propylene glycol—that are meant for use with shaving powder. The cream contains mineral oil and menthol to soothe and cool the face, and both products are widely available in drugstores. They're also priced very reasonably, and the difference between them boils down to one being a blue liquid and the other a cream.

There is an abundance of medium-priced aftershave lotions, all very much the same. Remember that you can read the ingredients for yourself on the labels these days. If you want something oily and soothing, look between the multisyllabic chemicals for ingredients like glycerine, lanolin, mineral oil, or propylene glycol. If you want a slap-in-the-face tingle from your aftershave, steer clear of the soothers and stick with high-alcohol formulas and those with salicylic acid. This last ingredient is a vigorous degreaser found in acne medicines, and it really smarts.

The Mennen Co. of Morristown, New Jersey, makes a number of old standbys, notably: MENNEN SKIN BRACER (with propylene glycol, plus, of all things, a little saccharin); MENNEN AFTA AFTER SHAVE SKIN CONDITIONER (which is alcohol plus triethanolamine, a lubricating substance that is also the basis of Neutrogena soap); and MENNEN MEDICATED FACE CONDITIONER (with salicylic acid and lots of alcohol; guaranteed to wake you up fast).

Shulton, Inc., in Clifton, New Jersey, makes several equally good products, such as OLD SPICE AFTER SHAVE SKIN CONDITIONER (with lanolin and only a third of the alcoholic content in the Mennen Medicated Face Conditioner above), OLD

SPICE AFTER SHAVE (with propylene glycol in the classic Old Spice bottle), and OLD SPICE MUSK FOR MEN AFTER SHAVE LOTION (which is the same as regular Old Spice, except for the scent). Remember to beware the Fresh Lime varieties of Old Spice because of the phototoxic characteristics of lime essence.

Fortunately, YARDLEY ORIGINAL AFTER SHAVE, which describes itself as "mature, accomplished and brisk when applied," also smells good and costs surprisingly little. The formula contains soothing glycerine, as does that of WOODBURY AFTER SHAVE (made by the famous Jergen hand-lotion people). Woodbury calls itself as "brisk as a mountain breeze," which is good to know in case Yardley isn't "accomplished" enough for you.

But, of course, all these products constitute the merest sampling of what's on the market. Especially in good department stores, there seems no end to aftershaves. If you're going to spend more than $1.50 to $2, I again urge you to consider cologne (see Chapter 3), which is often cheaper and smells just as good. JEAN NATÉ FOR MEN AFTER SHAVE is probably the least expensive department-store aftershave, and EAU SAUVAGE by Christian Dior is about the costliest. I personally love the scent of Eau Sauvage and let that be widely known each Christmastime. However, I always ask for the cologne. A list of good department-store aftershave lotions, most of which also come in cologne form, includes ARAMIS (in a half-dozen permutations of basically the same product), CHANEL, BRITISH STERLING, BRAVURA, ENGLISH LEATHER, KANON, BRAGGI, PIERRE CARDIN, ROYAL COPENHAGEN, etc. There is no great difference—at least medically speaking—among these.

Depilatories and Epilators

Depilatories are chemical concoctions usually based on sodium thioglycolate, a substance that softens hair so much it can literally be wiped off the skin. Epilators are physical methods for plucking hairs from their follicles. Wax is the most common epilator. Perma Tweez, a small home hair-removal appliance described in Chapter 15, is also an epilator.

Let's start with depilatories, which do have major drawbacks. The least of these is the smell, which is awful. The manufacturers disguise it as best they can, but. . . . Depilatories can also irritate the skin. Again, the makers add soothing ingredients, like mineral oil, to mitigate the harsh thioglycolate, but the potential for irritation is high. Last and worst is the high incidence of sensitization and allergic reaction to any of a depilatory's many strong ingredients.

Depilatories are mainly for women—even though men's shaving powder is really a depilatory, too. I see many women in my practice who suffer from skin irritations, stemming usually from thioglycolate. Depilatories advertise themselves as the feminine way to remove hair, but surveys show that only 5% of women who keep their legs and underarms free of hair use them. The rest shave.

Depilatories are slow and messy and even expensive. Smoothing a pair of legs sometimes costs nearly $1 with a hair-removal cream or spray, as compared to

SHAVING AND HAIR REMOVAL

a fraction of that cost with a razor. However, depilatories rarely do any serious physical harm. They are also a godsend to women with varicose veins.

Before you use a depilatory, you must put a dab on your skin a full day before use. This is a "sensitization test" to see whether or not you'll have an adverse reaction to the chemicals. Assuming your sensitization test is negative, apply the product as directed, wait the required number of minutes, then test a small area to see if the hair wipes easily away. If it doesn't, wait a few minutes more and test again. If it does, remove the product with water or a wet cloth. For application to face or underarms, spray or pour the product onto the fingers and apply.

Whitehall Laboratories in New York City makes what I believe is the least irritating depilatory. Marketed variously as SPRAY NEET HAIR REMOVER, NEET CREAM HAIR REMOVER, and NEET LOTION HAIR REMOVER, it contains thioglycolate and perfume, with mineral oil and paraffin in the spray and lotion forms, and with chalk and simethicone (a lubricating substance) in the cream. I also like the various forms of NAIR, a product of Carter-Wallace, and NUDIT, made by Helena Rubinstein. In addition to the standard thioglycolate and perfume, Nair contains light mineral oil and petrolatum, both oily and soothing substances. Nudit comes with a specially boxed brush and bottle for applying the cream to the face, and contains extracts of sweet birch and chamomile as well as chalk. Regular Nudit cream for the face contains petrolatum, mineral oil, and isopropyl palmitate, all of which are oily and soothing. The Nudit leg formula also comes in an aerosol spray.

There are numerous other depilatories—for example, SCHOLL LEG HAIR REMOVER—that do the job approximately as well as the products above, but I prefer Neet to any other. Actually, for legs and underarms, an electric razor (see the evaluations that follow) is a much better idea. That's because it's the least abrasive—if not the closest—form of removing hair from these sensitive areas.

On to epilators, my favorite of which is ZIP DEPILATORY WAX. This is a home waxing kit with detailed instructions on how to melt the wax cubes, apply the molten wax to the skin in an even coating, and remove the cooled wax together with the hair. Wax just provides a convenient handle with which to yank hairs out of the follicles. Like shaving or using a depilatory, waxing only temporarily removes hair. Neither depilatories nor epilators affect the follicles that grow hair. It is therefore doubtful that any of these products has a long-term effect on rate and strength of future hair growth—despite the manufacturers' claims.

Another product, similar to Zip, is NEW ORGANIC HAIR REMOVER STRIPS. These are like wax, except you don't have to melt cubes or apply hot wax to the skin. Instead, the strips come in the box and are ready to be pressed onto the skin, then yanked off with a sharp, quick movement. They're a lot less trouble, but not quite as thorough as Zip.

Again, there are many other waxing preparations—DOROTHY GRAY WAX, for example, which is a good luxury choice available in department stores—and they all work on the same yank-it-out principle. Except for Dorothy Gray, most waxes are sold in drugstores.

Electric Razors

There's a welter of disagreement about electric razors. Some people find them less irritating; some people find them more irritating; I think they're basically unnecessary. But, although I recommend regular razors for faces, I must admit that electrics are often much more convenient for legs and underarms.

Wherever you use an electric, the shave will not be as close as it will be with a blade and shaving cream. This is true of both men's and women's electrics. In fact, whatever is true of men's electrics is also true of women's. The machines work on identical principles, and only the size varies.

There are three basic design approaches to electric shavers. My favorite is the rotary head, on which three spinning cutting edges are screened by the same number of floating circular guard disks. Shavers of this design—notably the NORELCO RECHARGEABLE TRIPLEHEADER III DELUXE 45 CT, the NORELCO RECHARGEABLE TRIPLE-HEADER VIP50, the NORELCO SPEEDSHAVER 11 20, the NORELCO TRIPLEHEADER III 35 T, and the LADY NORELCO 20 L—give the closest shaves with the least pulling, nicking, and irritation. Rotary-head Norelcos are also relatively quiet and are easy to hold.

There is practically no end to the extra features available on electric shavers. They range from retractable trimmers, to special voltage selectors, to extra-durable travel cases, to electric wall-charge converters, to charge-indicator lights, etc. I think the fewer the frills, the better the buy. The Norelco Speedshaver 11 20 and the Lady Norelco 20 L are basic rotary-head models with the best (i.e. lowest) prices.

Other electric shavers have cutting edges that slide back and forth beneath protective guards that are either curved or flat. I much prefer the Norelcos above and give a blanket second place rating to the following: REMINGTON LB30 LEKTRO BLADE SHAVER; REMINGTON LBX LEKTRO BLADE SHAVER; LADY REMINGTON LR70M; LADY SHAVEX 1700; SCHICK STAYSHARP SS11; and PANASONIC ES306 DURANGO.

I do *not* recommend the following shavers for the reasons noted: RONSON 100 XL (very hard to clean); SUNBEAM SHAVEMASTER 5671 (very noisy and hard to clean); SHAVEX CORDLESS RECHARGEABLE XL400 (noisy, irritating, and hard to clean); LADY SUNBEAM TWIN-HEAD LS9 (poor shave); LADY SCHICK SHAVING WAND (convenient to use, but gives a mediocre shave); the JEWEL BY LADY SCHICK (lots of noise and vibration); NORELCO LADYSHAVE HP2108 (a slow and uneven shaver); and the REMINGTON PRINCESS CL50 (awkward to hold and doesn't give a close shave).

Electric shavers are usually list-priced between $20 and $60, but the price you actually pay can vary widely from store to store. You've got to comparison shop; there's lots of competition.

People have very different ideas of comfort, convenience, and just what constitutes a good shave. It's very possible you won't like a shaver that most other people find very good. Which is why I strongly urge you to purchase your shaver from a dealer who'll give you the right to exchange it if necessary.

SHAVING AND HAIR REMOVAL

An electric shaver is also something of a precision instrument. If you buy one, you're obligating yourself to regular cleaning, blade replacement (at $4 to $6 every six months to a year), and general caution. Few electric razors can survive a fall on the bathroom floor without extensive and possibly expensive damage. Be prepared for this maintenance. Without it, your shaver will not shave well.

CHAPTER 3

Perfumes and Colognes for Men and Women

If you're like most people, you're probably not really sure what to buy when you go shopping for a scent. Should you get perfume, or cologne, or eau de toilette, or eau de perfume, or perfume concentrate, or spray concentrate, or *what?* There are so many different forms of packaging that everybody's just got to be confused. The difference between all these forms simply lies in the proportion of essence (the stuff that makes it smell) to alcohol. However, there are no government regulations dictating how much essence must be contained in the bottle to call it one thing rather than something else. That's why most shoppers rarely know exactly what they're getting.

What's worse, scents for both sexes are *expensive.* There is some justification for the high cost of many scents. The art of the perfumer is a complicated one; some scents have as many as two hundred separate ingredients. These include leaves, roots, flowers, fruits, needles, gums, ambergris, distilled essences, musk, lots of alcohol, and a host of chemicals.

Good perfumes typically contain about twenty-four ounces of perfume essence per gallon of alcohol. Cologne usually contains somewhere between three and six ounces of the same essence per gallon of alcohol. Toilet water (or "eau de toilette," if you will) is for all intents and purposes identical to cologne (sometimes it's a little stronger). Aftershave lotion for men (described in Chapter 2) contains less essence per volume than does perfume for women. But aftershaves have more essence per volume than men's colognes. Both men's and women's colognes are equally strong, meaning they have approximately the same ratio of essence to alcohol.

Be you man or woman, you are more sensible to use cologne rather than perfume or aftershave. Cologne is not only cheaper, but, because it's meant to be liberally splashed onto the body, it permits a far greater area of skin coverage. This in turn permits a more effective rate of dissolution into the air around you.

Perfume, by contrast, is meant to be applied sparingly on spots at the wrist, behind the ears, and around the neck. Although it is far more concentrated than cologne, its scent actually lasts *no longer* than that of cologne. This is because

PERFUMES AND COLOGNES

perfume is applied to so small an area of skin; the dissolution rate correlates directly to surface area covered, as well as to rate of perspiration and the temperature of the room you're in.

Aftershave is marketed as if it were meant to be used on the face only. Since it's about the least soothing thing you could possibly apply to a freshly shaved face, the only justification for using it has to be its scent. You'll get a better dissolution rate—at a better price—by splashing cologne freely on the face as well as on the body, than you will by simply applying aftershave to the face. Some men are reluctant to use cologne on the chest, arms, throat, and face lest they be thought effeminate. This is simply an irrational prejudice, especially among men who already use scented aftershaves.

No matter what form of scent you fancy, you should avoid application to areas of the skin that will be exposed to sunlight for any length of time. Many perfume essences are photosensitizing, meaning they'll cause a rash in the presence of sunlight. If not a rash, sometimes you'll just get a bad sunburn. Although not everybody suffers from this photosensitizing phenomenon, enough people do for there to be a special medical name for it. "Berloque dermatitis," as it's called, often appears around the necks of women who pat on their perfume then lie down in the sun by the pool. *Berloque* means "necklace" in French, and the lesions resulting from the sun and the perfume do in fact look like a necklace.

Now then, as to what scent is right for you—well, that's not an easy question. What's more, the same scent smells different on different human bodies. Then there's the question of the rip-off scents, the ones that claim to smell exactly like the high-priced models at a fraction of the cost. If you're in love with a certain scent, if the prestige associated with the packaging matters naught, and if you're buying for yourself (as opposed to getting a gift for someone), then by all means try the rip-offs. They are in no way medically inferior to the originals, nor are any that I've encountered dangerous. If your own nose can't tell the difference, go ahead and save the money.

Whether you go with one of the rip-offs (which advertise regularly in the backs of magazines and in the newspapers) or stay with the brand-name originals, you're still buying a blind item. The merit of any scent rests totally on a rather subtle combination of its impact on your nose (and the noses of others) together with the image its advertisers have managed to implant in your subconscious. If there is no acceptable rip-off available for the scent you like, then you'll just have to pay the price, no matter how exorbitant. And remember, you'll smell more of whatever it is you're wearing if you use it in the cologne form.

One of the most ridiculous aspects of the perfume game is the rigid segregation between men's and women's scents. Everything—from advertising, to nomenclature to packaging—strives to project an image that is distinctly *either* masculine *or* feminine. I think this stems purely from a reluctance on the part of manufacturers to contradict presumed public attitudes concerning masculinity and femininity. But it doesn't take much liberation to realize that there is nothing inherently "masculine" or "feminine" about a scent.

Recently an interesting study illustrated this point. Cited in *Cosmetics, Science and Technology* by M. S. Balsan and Edward Sargarin (John Wiley & Sons, 1974), the study involved a single colorless scent and a wide sample of human subjects who were asked to describe it. Glass vials of the scent were backed with different-colored strips giving the appearance of different-colored liquids. The test subjects believed that they were being given different scents to evaluate. When the scent was backed with a blue strip, it was invariably described as masculine and potent; when the same scent was backed with magenta, it was described as sensual; and if the strip was yellow, it was described as sweet and probably expensive!

This test shows how an apparently straightforward evaluation can be subtly influenced by psychological factors. The smell of the test scent was neither the sole nor even the most critical factor governing its appeal. By extrapolation, there should be no reason for women not to enjoy men's colognes—particularly since men's scents are cheaper than women's. In fact, many women do wear colognes—particularly Old Spice and Canoe—that are exclusively designed and packaged for men.

All colognes, perfumes, aftershaves, toilet waters, etc., containing the amount of alcohol they do, are drying to the skin. If you have dry skin, you're better off not to splash alcoholic cologne or toilet water all over yourself. You can either use the more potent perfume form in sparing drops, or mix those drops with a moisturizing cream like Nivea. This is an excellent solution, especially for chronically dry-skinned older women.

There's also the problem of allergies. Given the many chemicals and extracts in perfume essence, there are bound to be some people who will break out in a rash from the application of almost any perfume. Oddly, allergic reactions are more common with more expensive scents. Some dermatologists believe the rashes are caused by essential oils frequently found in quality perfumes; these are "fumo-coumarin" and "oil of bergamot." Unfortunately, these ingredients are not listed on labels. But if you have a reaction to your perfume, this is probably the reason, and there's nothing to do but change scents. Remember that these substances are found in expensive scents, so don't expect to avoid them just by spending more money.

Berloque dermatitis, the photosensitive reaction discussed above, has an unfortunate tendency to develop "postinflammatory hyperpigmentation." Stated simply, this is an unattractive darkening of the skin that appears on the site of a rash after it has otherwise cleared up. It can best be avoided by (1) immediately discontinuing use of any scent at the first sign of a rash; (2) treating the rash

PERFUMES AND COLOGNES

immediately with the soothing compress described on page 9, and (3) *never* wearing perfume on skin that will be exposed to bright sunshine.

Dr. Alex Fisher, one of the world's authorities on contact dermatitis, has recently discovered what he calls the "quenching phenomenon." Dr. Fisher found that people who are allergic to certain essential oils are very often *not* allergic to them when the oils are sufficiently diluted with alcohol. It's as if the potential for the allergic reaction were literally quenched by the alcohol. This means that many people can wear a cologne without any adverse effects, even when the perfume form of the same scent causes an allergic reaction. This is yet another reason to buy colognes instead of perfumes, since, statistically, colognes pose a lesser danger of provoking adverse skin reactions.

The scent of a body that's been washed and perfumed is still greatly influenced by heat and humidity. Hot weather makes perfumes dissipate quickly. Humidity makes them smell more potent. Be particularly careful in humid weather not to overdo perfume or cologne application lest the smell be too pungent.

What follows are price analysis charts that profile a wide sample of available fragrances as to price, size, and packaging. Though these charts are divided by "men's" and "women's" products, these are manufacturer's distinctions. Let me again emphasize the silliness of this division and urge all readers to at least sample other scents regardless of the "sexual orientation" of the packaging. Please note that Men's Colognes, listed in the first chart that follows, have by far the best (i.e. lowest) prices. In general, drugstores will carry most colognes and toilet waters, whereas, to be sure of getting full-strength perfume, you'll usually have to go to a big department store.

Women's Perfumes, which follow, have the highest prices and the tiniest volume—even higher and tinier in atomizer form. I seriously question whether their potency is worth the extra price in practical terms. Colognes and toilet waters, profiled further below, simply dispel more scent per dollar spent.

As noted earlier, the United States government exercises no controls whatsoever on the use of the words "cologne," "toilet water," and "perfume." Generally speaking, cologne is slightly weaker than toilet water—but not always. Some manufacturers offer their scents in so many different forms that only the prices will give you a hint as to which contain more or less essence.

This lack of standardized terms has caused a confusing proliferation of labels like "100 strength," "80 strength," "concentrated cologne," "eau de cologne," "eau de perfume" and so on. A rapid glance at the prices below, however, will make it immediately clear that colognes are much much cheaper than their parent perfumes. And, frankly, assuming your goal is to impart to the body a subtle scent, you can really do it much more cheaply and—yes—thoroughly with cologne. The women's colognes that follow may be a bargain when compared to women's perfume prices, but they're very high compared to the prices of men's colognes. Fortunately, almost all these products (men's included) come in at least one tiny bottle.

MEN'S COLOGNES

SUPER BODY CONSUMER SURVEY CHART #1: MEN'S COLOGNES*

Brand Name	Manufacturer	Price of 4-oz. sample bottle	Additional sizes and forms
DELUXE (SAMPLE BOTTLE OVER $16)			
Brut 33	Fabergé, Inc.	$24 (for 3.5 ozs.)	nonaerosol spray and special musk cologne scent
Yatagan	Caron Parfums	$16	2- and 6-oz. bottles
HIGH PRICED (SAMPLE BOTTLE $12.50 TO $15)			
Paco Rabanne	Puig/Barcelona, Inc.	$15	2-, 8-, 16-, 32-oz. bottles; 3-oz. spray
Grey Flannel	Geoffrey Beene	$15	8-oz. bottle; 4-oz. spray
Chromatics	Aramis, Inc.	$15	spray concentrate and splash forms
Capucci "Pour Homme"	Parfums Capucci	$14.50	2- and 8-oz. bottles; 3½-oz. spray
Herbal	Aramis, Inc.	$12.50	spray concentrate and spray concentrate forms
MEDIUM PRICED (SAMPLE BOTTLE $8.50 TO $11.50)			
1–12	Halston	$11.50	8-oz. bottle
Z-14	Halston	$11.50	8-oz. bottle
Macho	Fabergé, Inc.	$11.50 (for 3.75 ozs.)	2-oz. bottle
Equipage	Parfums Hermés	$11.50	2-, 8-, 16-, 32-oz. bottles; 4-oz. atomizer
Bill Blass	Revlon, Inc.	$11.50	"60-strength" 4-oz. bottle; 3.5-oz. "100-strength" spray
Pierre Cardin	Jacqueline Cochran, Inc.	$11	2- and 8-oz. bottles; 2.5-oz. spray
Givenchy Gentleman	Parfums Givenchy, Inc.	$11	2- and 7.3-oz. bottles; 3½-oz. spray
Yves Saint Laurent for Men	Lanvin-Charles of the Ritz	$11	8-oz. bottle; 2- and 4-oz. atomizers; ¼-oz. concentrated pocket spray
Acqua di Selva	Victor of Milano	$11	in several sizes up to 14 ozs.; 1.9- and 3.5-oz. atomizers

* Survey based on 4-oz. sample bottle. All prices subject to change.

Continued

PERFUMES AND COLOGNES

Cont.

Brand Name	Manufacturer	Price of 4-oz. sample bottle	Additional sizes and forms
Eau Sauvage	Christian Dior	$11 (for 3.7 ozs.)	1.9-, 7.5-, 15-, 32-oz. bottles; 2- and 4-oz. atomizers.
Aramis	Aramis, Inc.	$10.50	2-, 8-, 16-, 32-oz. bottles; 2- and 4-oz. sprays; 2-oz. "fortified" cologne and spray
Canoe	Dana Perfumes	$10	"eau de cologne" form up to 32.4 ozs.; 4-oz. spray
Patrick	Patrick Ltd.	$10	
Braggi	Charles Revson	$10	2.9- and 10-oz. bottles; 3-oz. spray
Royal Copenhagen	Swank, Inc.	$10	2-, 6-, 8-oz. bottles; 2- and 4-oz. sprays; special "musk" scented cologne and spray
Kanon	Scannon Ltd.	$9.50	7-oz. bottle
Lenel for Men	Lenel Toiletries	$9	½-oz. bottle
Chaz	Revlon, Inc.	$9	2.25- and 8-oz. bottles; 1- and 3-oz. sprays
Pino Silvestre	Int'l Perfumes Ltd.	$8.50	⅓-oz. "perfume"; wide range of cologne sizes up to 21 ozs.; 2.5-oz. spray
Pour un Homme	Caron Parfums	$8.50	5.75-, 8-, 13.5-oz. bottles

INEXPENSIVE (SAMPLE BOTTLE $4 TO $7)

Brand Name	Manufacturer	Price of 4-oz. sample bottle	Additional sizes and forms
Chanel for Men	Chanel, Inc.	$7.50	3- and 8-oz. bottles; 3-oz. spray
Jean Marie Forina	Roger & Gallet	$7	3.4-, 6.7-, 13.5-, 27-oz. decorative bottles; 2- and 4-oz. sprays
Musk Oil for Men	Jovan, Inc.	$7	½-oz. bottle; 3-oz. spray
Ginseng for Men	Jovan, Inc.	$7	½-oz. bottle
Monsieur Houbigant	Houbigant, Inc.	$6.50	8-oz. bottle; 3-oz. spray

Continued

WOMEN'S PERFUMES

Cont.

Brand Name	Manufacturer	Price of 4-oz. sample bottle	Additional sizes and forms
Monsieur Houbigant Musk	Houbigant, Inc.	$6	2- and 8-oz. bottles; 5.5-oz. spray; ½-oz. oil
Caesar	Paris Presents	$6.50	8- and 16-oz. bottles
British Sterling	Speidel Textron, Inc.	$6	2- and 5.7-oz. bottles; 3.5-oz. spray
Mon Triomphe	J. B. Williams Co., Inc.	$6	3-oz. spray; 4-oz. "Musk Plus Cologne"
Jade East	Swank, Inc.	$5	2- and 6-oz. bottles; 4-oz. spray; 4-oz. "musk oil cologne"
Ginseng for Men	MEM Co., Inc.	$5 (for 5 ozs.)	½-oz. bottle
Drift	MEM Co., Inc.	$4.50 (for 3.75 ozs.)	7.75-oz. bottle
English Leather	MEM Co., Inc.	$4.50	8- and 16-oz. bottles
Yardley Original Cologne	Yardley of London	$4 (for 4.12 ozs.)	
Old Spice Cologne for Men	Shulton, Inc.	$3.50 (for 4.75 ozs.)	9.5-oz. bottle; "fresh lime" scent in 4.75- and 9.5-oz. bottles

SUPER BODY CONSUMER SURVEY CHART #2: WOMEN'S PERFUMES**

Brand Name	Manufacturer	Price of ¼-oz. sample bottle	Price /oz.	Additional sizes and forms
DELUXE (SAMPLE BOTTLE OVER $23)				
Joy	Jean Patou	$35	$100	in many different sizes; 1-oz. Baccarat crystal bottle for $225; ⅓-oz. spray
HIGH PRICED (SAMPLE BOTTLE $18 TO $23)				
Chloe	Parfums Lagerfeld	$22.50	$60	½-, 1-, 2-oz. bottles; ⅓-oz. spray "vaporiseur"
Ciara	Charles Revson	$20	$65	½-oz. bottle; ⅓-oz. spray
Cerissa	Charles Revson	$20	$65	½-oz. bottle

** Survey based on ¼-oz. sample perfume bottle. All prices subject to change.

Continued

PERFUMES AND COLOGNES

Cont.

Brand Name	Manufacturer	Price of ¼-oz. sample bottle	Price /oz.	Additional sizes and forms
Norell	Norell Perfumes	$20	$65	½-, 1-, 2-oz. bottles; ⅕-oz. spray
Givenchy III	Parfums Givenchy	$18.50	$55	½-, 1-, 2-oz. bottles; ⅕-oz. "mist"; .15-oz. solid perfume
Calandre by Paco Rabanne	Puig/ Barcelona, Inc.	$18	$55	½-, 1-, 2-oz. bottles; ¼- and 1-oz. sprays
MEDIUM HIGH PRICED (SAMPLE BOTTLE $12 TO $16.50)				
L'Interdit	Parfums Givenchy, Inc.	$16.50	$48	½-, 1-, 1⅘-oz. bottles; ⅕-oz. mist
Le De	Parfums Givenchy, Inc.	$16.50	$48	½-, 1-, 1⅘-, 3⅔-oz. bottles; ⅕-oz. mist
Y	Yves Saint Laurent	$16	$45	½-, 1-, 2-, 4-oz. bottles; ¼-oz. atomizer; 1-oz. aerosol
Ode	Guerlain, Inc.	$16	—	½-oz. bottle
Miss Dior	Christian Dior	$15.50 (for .2 oz.)	$50	½- and 1-oz. bottles; .4- and .8-oz. atomizers
Diorissimo	Christian Dior	$15.50 (for .2 oz.)	$50	½- and 1-oz. bottles; .4- and .8-oz. atomizers
Diorella	Christian Dior	$15.50	$50	½- and 1-oz. bottles; ¼-oz. spray
Maja	Myurgia Perfumes, Inc.	$15	$40	½- and 1-oz. bottles; ⅐-oz. perfume "miniature"; 3½-oz. perfume "cream"
Caleche	Parfums Hermés	$15	$45	½-, 1-, 2-, 4-oz. bottles; 1- and 4-oz. "deluxe" bottles; ⅕-oz. atomizer
Infini	Caron Parfums	$15	$45	½-, 1-, 2-oz. bottles; ⅙-oz. spray
Cabochard	Parfums Gres	$15	$45	½-, 1-, 2-, 4-oz. bottles; ¼- and 1-oz. sprays
Farouche	Nini Ricci	$14.50	$45	⅙-, ½-, 1-oz. bottles; ¼-oz. spray
Chamade	Guerlain, Inc.	$14	$46	½-, 1-, 2-oz. bottles; ¼-oz. spray

Continued

WOMEN'S PERFUMES

Cont.

Brand Name	Manufacturer	Price of ¼-oz. sample bottle	Price /oz.	Additional sizes and forms
Chant d'Arômes	Guerlain, Inc.	$14	$46	½-, 1-, 2-oz. bottles; ¼-oz. spray
Shalimar	Guerlain, Inc.	$14	$46	⅓-, ½-, 1-, 2-, 4-oz. bottles; ¼-oz. spray
Femme	Parfums Rochas	$14	$50	½-, 1-, 2-oz. bottles; ⅕-, ¼-, 1⅙-oz. atomizers
Madame Rochas	Parfums Rochas	$14	$50	⅙-, ½-, 1-, 2-oz. bottles; ⅕-, ¼-, 1⅙-oz. atomizers
Diagonal	Puig/Barcelona, Inc.	$14	$37	½- and 1-oz. bottles; ¼- and ½-oz. sprays
L'Air du Temps	Nina Ricci	$13.50	$40	⅙-, ⅕-, ½-, 1-, 2-, 3.3-, 8-oz. bottles in many decorative shapes; ⅕-, ¼-, ½-, ¾-oz. sprays
Capricci	Nina Ricci	$13.50	$40	⅙-, ⅕-, ½-, ⁶⁄₇-, 1-, 1½-oz. bottles in many decorative shapes; ⅕-oz. spray
Bellodgia	Caron Parfums	$13.50	$45	½-, 1-, 2-oz. bottles; ⅙-oz. spray
Fleurs de Rocaille	Caron Parfums	$13.50	$45	½-, 1-, 2-oz. bottles; ⅙-oz. spray
Nuit de Noel	Caron Parfums	$13.50	$45	½-, 1-, 2-oz. bottles; ⅙-oz. spray
Narcisse Noir	Caron Parfums	$13.50	$45	½-, 1-, 2-oz. bottles; ¼-oz. spray
Le Muguet De Bonheur	Caron Parfums	$13.50	$45	½-, 1-, 2-oz. bottles; ¼-oz. spray
Tabac Blond	Caron Parfums	$13.50	$45	½-, 1-, 2-oz. bottles; ¼-oz. spray
Les Pois De Senteur	Caron Parfums	$13.50	$45	½-, 1-, 2-oz. bottles; ¼-oz. spray
L'Heure Bleue	Guerlain, Inc.	$13	$32	½-, 1-, 2-oz. bottles; ¼-oz. spray
Mitsouko	Guerlain, Inc.	$13	$32	½-, 1-, 2-oz. bottles; ¼-oz. spray
Vol De Nuit	Guerlain, Inc.	$13	$32	½-, 1-, 2-oz. bottles; ¼-oz. spray

Continued

PERFUMES AND COLOGNES

Cont.

Brand Name	Manufacturer	Price of ¼-oz. sample bottle	Price /oz.	Additional sizes and forms
Chanel No. 5	Chanel, Inc.	$12.50	$45	⅓-, ½-, 1-, 2-, 4-oz. bottles; ¼-, 1.5-oz. sprays
Chanel No. 19	Chanel, Inc.	$12.50	$45	⅓-, ½-, 1-, 2-, 4-oz. bottles; ¼-, 1.5-oz. sprays
Chanel No. 22	Chanel, Inc.	$12.50	$45	⅓-, ½-, 1-, 2-, 4-oz. bottles; ¼-oz. spray
Arpege	Lanvin-Charles of the Ritz	$12.50	$45	⅛-, ½-, 1-oz. bottles; deluxe 1-oz. sphere bottle; ¼-oz. mist
My Sin	Lanvin-Charles of the Ritz	$12.50	$45	⅛-, ½-, 1-oz. bottles
Aviance	Prince Matchabelli	$12.50	—	⅕-oz. spray; and 1-oz. "creme perfume"
Nuance	Coty	$12.50	$40	1-oz. bottle; .17-oz. spray
Replique	Parfums Raphael	$12	$35	½-, 1-, 2-oz. bottles; ¼-oz. spray
Cie	Contemporary Fragrance Group	$12	—	⅓-oz. atomizer

MEDIUM PRICED (SAMPLE BOTTLE $8 TO $11)

Brand Name	Manufacturer	Price of ¼-oz. sample bottle	Price /oz.	Additional sizes and forms
Chantilly	Houbigant, Inc.	$10	$33	.13-, ½-, 1-oz. bottles; ¼-oz. spray
Rive Gauche	Lanvin-Charles of the Ritz	$22 (for ½ oz.)	$38	1-oz. bottle; ¼-oz. spray; ¼- and 4-oz. "solid perfume"

INEXPENSIVE (SAMPLE BOTTLE $2 TO $6)

Brand Name	Manufacturer	Price of ¼-oz. sample bottle	Price /oz.	Additional sizes and forms
Twenty Carats	Dana Perfumes	$6 (specially priced ⅓-oz. spray)	$35	1-oz. bottle; ⅓-oz. spray
Jicky	Guerlain, Inc.		$23	
Blue Carnation	Roger & Gallet	$5 (for ⅛ oz.)	$28	½- and 1-oz. bottles; ¼-oz. spray; ½- and 1¼-oz. "dry perfume"

Continued

WOMEN'S PERFUMES

Cont.

Brand Name	Manufacturer	Price of ¼-oz. sample bottle	Price /oz.	Additional sizes and forms
Charlie	Revlon, Inc.	$4.50 (specially priced ⅜-oz. bottle)	$35	½- and 1-oz. bottles; ⅓- and ½-oz. sprays
Jontue	Revlon, Inc.	$4.50 (for ⅜ oz.)	N.A.	
Mink & Pearls	Jovan, Inc.	$2 (for ⅛ oz.)	N.A.	⅕-oz. "solid perfume"
Madame Jovan	Jovan, Inc.	$2 (for ⅛ oz.)	N.A.	⅓-oz. bottle; ⅕-oz. "solid perfume"
Ginseng	Jovan, Inc.	$2 (for ⅛ oz.)	N.A.	⅓-oz. bottle; ⅕-oz. "solid perfume"
Musk Oil	Jovan, Inc.	$2 (for ⅛ oz.)	N.A.	⅓-oz. bottle; ⅕-oz. "perfume wand"; ⅕-oz. "solid perfume"

SUPER BODY CONSUMER SURVEY CHART #3: WOMEN'S COLOGNES AND TOILET WATERS***

DELUXE (SAMPLE BOTTLE OVER $12.50)

Brand Name	Manufacturer	Price of 2-oz. sample bottle	Additional sizes and forms
Eau de Joy	Jean Patou	$29 (for 1½ oz.)	1-, 3-, 6-oz. bottles; 1½-oz. spray; 2-oz. atomizer aerosol

HIGH PRICED (SAMPLE BOTTLE $9 TO $12.50)

Brand Name	Manufacturer	Price of 2-oz. sample bottle	Additional sizes and forms
Chloe Eau de Toilette	Parfums Lagerfeld	$12.50	4- and 8-oz. bottles; 3-oz. atomizer
Ciara 100 strength concentrated cologne	Charles Revson	$12 (for 2⅛ oz.)	"80 strength" concentrated cologne
Norell Cologne	Norell Perfumes	$12 (for 2¼ oz.)	4- and 8-oz. bottles; 1¼- and 2¼-oz. sprays; .3-oz. "spray concentrate"

*** Survey based on 2-oz. sample bottle. All prices subject to change.

Continued

PERFUMES AND COLOGNES

Cont.

Brand Name	Manufacturer	Price of 2-oz. sample bottle	Additional sizes and forms
Diorella Eau de toilette	Christian Dior	$11	4-oz. bottle; 2- and 4-oz. atomizer; lesser strength "eau de cologne"
Y Eau de toilette	Yves Saint Laurent	$10	4-, 8-, 16-oz. bottles; 2- and 2½-oz. sprays; stronger 2¼-oz. "parfum de toilette"
Cerissa Concentrated Cologne	Charles Revson	$10 (for 2⅛ oz.)	3½-oz. bottle
Eau de Calandre	Puig/Barcelona, Inc.	$10	4-, 8-, 16-oz. bottles; 3-oz. spray
Givenchy III Eau de toilette	Parfums Givenchy, Inc.	$9.50	4- and 8-oz. bottles; 2- and 3½-oz. sprays
Ultima Eau de perfume spray	Charles Revson	$8.50	3¾-oz. spray
Caleche Eau de toilette	Parfums Hermés	$8.50	4- and 8-oz. bottles; 2 oz. atomizer
Infini Parfum de toilette	Caron Parfums	$8.50	4-oz. bottle; 2½-oz. "parfum de toilette" spray; weaker 2¼-oz. "parfum de cologne" spray
Bellodgia Parfum de toilette	Caron Parfums	$8.50	4-oz. bottle; 2½-oz. "parfum de toilette" spray; weaker 2¼-oz. "parfum de cologne" spray
Fleurs de Rocaille/ Parfum de toilette	Caron Parfums	$8.50	4-oz. bottle; 2½-oz. "parfum de toilette" spray; weaker 2¼-oz. "parfum de cologne" spray
Nuit de Noel Parfum de toilette	Caron Parfums	$8.50	4-oz. bottle; 2½-oz. "parfum de toilette" spray; weaker 2¼-oz. "parfum de cologne" spray

Continued

WOMEN'S COLOGNES

Cont.

Brand Name	Manufacturer	Price of 2-oz. sample bottle	Additional sizes and forms
Narcisse Noir Parfum de toilette	Caron Parfums	$8.50	2¼-oz. "parfum de cologne" spray
Le Muguet de Bonheur Parfum de toilette	Caron Parfums	$8.50	
Tabac Blond Parfum de toilette	Caron Parfums	$8.50	
Les Pois de Senteur Parfum de toilette	Caron Parfums	$8.50	
Chamade Cologne	Guerlain, Inc.	$10 (for 3 oz.)	6-oz. bottle; stronger 3-oz. "toilet water spray"
Chant D'Aromes Cologne	Guerlain, Inc.	$10 (for 3 oz.)	6-oz. bottle; stronger 3-oz. "toilet water spray"
Mitsouko Cologne	Guerlain, Inc.	$10 (for 3 oz.)	6-oz. bottle; stronger 3-oz. "toilet water spray"
Vol de Nuit Cologne	Guerlain, Inc.	$10 (for 3 oz.)	6-oz. bottle; stronger 3-oz. "toilet water spray"
Shalimar Cologne	Guerlain, Inc.	$10 (for 3 oz.)	6-oz. bottle; 3-oz. cologne atomizer; stronger 3-oz. "toilet water"; 3-oz. "toilet water spray"
L'Heure Bleue Cologne	Guerlain, Inc.	$10 (for 3 oz.)	6-oz. bottle; 2½- and 3-oz. cologne atomizers; stronger 3-oz. "toilet water"; 3-oz. "toilet water spray"
Jicky Toilet Water	Guerlain, Inc.	$12 (for 3 oz.)	

Continued

PERFUMES AND COLOGNES

Cont.

Brand Name	Manufacturer	Price of 2-oz. sample bottle	Additional sizes and forms
Chanel No. 5 Eau de toilette	Chanel, Inc.	$8	4- and 8-oz. bottles; weaker 2-, 4-, 8-oz. bottles of "cologne"; 1½- and 3-oz. "spray cologne"
Chanel No. 19 Eau de toilette	Chanel, Inc.	$8	4-, 8-, 16-oz. bottles; weaker 2-, 4-, 8-oz. "eau de cologne; 1½-oz. "spray cologne"
Diagonal Eau de toilette	Puig/Barcelona, Inc.	$8	4- and 8-oz. bottles; 2½-oz. spray
Arpege Eau liquid cologne	Lanvin-Charles of the Ritz	$8	4- and 8-oz. bottles; 2- and 4-oz. sprays
My Sin Eau liquid cologne	Lanvin-Charles of the Ritz	$8	4- and 8-oz. bottles; 2- and 4-oz. sprays
Le De Eau de toilette	Parfums Givenchy, Inc.	$8	3.3-, 7.3-, 15-oz. bottles; 2-oz. "eau de perfume"; 3-oz. "eau de toilette" spray
L'Interdit Eau de toilette	Parfums Givenchy, Inc.	$8	3.3-, 7.3-, 15-oz. bottles; 2-oz. "eau de perfume"; 3-oz. "eau de toilette" spray
Cabochard Eau de toilette	Parfums Gres	$8	4-, 8-, 16-oz. bottles; 2.3-, 3.3-, 4-oz. sprays
Madame Rochas Cologne regular	Parfums Rochas	$7	4- and 7-oz. bottles; 2- and 4-oz. atomizers
Femme Cologne regular	Parfums Rochas	$7	4- and 7-oz. bottles; 2- and 4-oz. atomizers
Miss Dior Eau de Cologne	Christian Dior	$7 (for 1.8 oz.)	3.6-oz. bottle; stronger 2- and 4-oz. "eau de toilette" atomizers; 1.8-, 3.6-, 7.2-oz. bottles of "eau de toilette"
Diorissimo Eau de cologne	Christian Dior	$7	3.6-oz. bottle; stronger 2- and 4-oz. "eau de toilette" atomizers; 1.8-, 3.6-, 7.2-oz. bottles of "eau de toilette"

Continued

WOMEN'S COLOGNES

Cont.

Brand Name	Manufacturer	Price of 2-oz. sample bottle	Additional sizes and forms
L'Air Du Temps Eau de toilette	Nina Ricci	$7 (for 1.7 oz.)	3.3-, 6.6-, 15-oz. bottles; 2-, 2½-, 3¾-oz. sprays
Capricci Eau de toilette	Nina Ricci	$7 (for 1.8 oz.)	3.3-oz. bottle; 2-, 2½-, 3¾-oz. spray
Farouche Eau de toilette	Nina Ricci	$7 (for 1.7 oz.)	3.3- and 6.6-oz. bottles; 2- and 3¾-oz. sprays
Crepe de Chine Eau de toilette Concentrate	House of Fragrance, Inc.	$6.50 (for 3 oz.)	4¼-oz. bottle; 1- and 3-oz. sprays; stronger 2-oz. "eau de parfum" spray
Mink & Pearls Cologne Concentrate spray	Jovan, Inc.	$4 (for ⅞ oz.)	
Madame Jovan Cologne Concentrate Spray	Jovan, Inc.	$4 (for ⅞ oz.)	2¼-oz. "cologne spray"; 2¼-oz. "eau de toilette" spray
Ginseng Cologne Concentrate Spray	Jovan, Inc.	$4 (for ⅞ oz.)	2-oz. "cologne spray"
Musk Oil Cologne Concentrate Spray	Jovan, Inc.	$4 (for ⅞ oz.)	2-oz. spray; 2-oz. "spray mist"

INEXPENSIVE (SAMPLE BOTTLE $4 TO $6)

Brand Name	Manufacturer	Price of 2-oz. sample bottle	Additional sizes and forms
Chanel No. 22 Eau de Cologne	Chanel, Inc.	$6	4-, 8-, 16-oz. bottles; 1½-oz. spray
Maja Cologne	Myurgia Perfumes, Inc.	$6 (for 1¾ oz.)	1-, 3½-, 7-, 14-oz. bottles; 2-, 3-, 4-oz. sprays
Chantilly Eau de toilette	Houbigant, Inc.	$6	4-oz. bottle; 1-, 2½-, 3.75-oz. sprays; stronger 2-oz. "parfum de toilette spray mist"
Charlie Cologne	Revlon, Inc.	$6 (for 3½ oz.)	8-, 16-oz. bottles; 2-, 2¼-oz. "concentrated cologne"; ½-, 2⅛-, 2¼-, 3½-oz. "concentrated cologne spray"

Continued

PERFUMES AND COLOGNES

Cont.

Brand Name	Manufacturer	Price of 2-oz. sample bottle	Additional sizes and forms
Replique Eau de toilette	Parfums Raphael	$5	4-oz. bottle; 1- and 3-oz. sprays
Rive Gauche Cologne	Lanvin-Charles of the Ritz	$9 (for 4 oz.)	8-oz. bottle; 4-oz. spray
Blue Carnation Eau de toilette	Roger & Gallet	$5	4-oz. bottle; 2- and 4-oz. sprays
Jean Naté Friction pour le bain	Lanvin-Charles of the Ritz	$3 (for 8 oz.)	16-, 32-, 128-oz. containers; 1-, 2-, 3-oz. sprays; 1¼-oz. "cologne stick"; 7-oz. "cologne cooler"; ½-oz. "essence of Naté perfume spray"
Cie Lavish Cologne	Contemporary Fragrance Group	$5 (for 4 oz.)	8-oz. bottle
Jontue Cologne	Revlon, Inc.	$5 (for 2½ oz.)	5-oz. bottle; ¾-, 1½-, 3-oz. sprays
Aviance Cologne	Prince Matchabelli	$5	4-oz. bottle; 1.7-, and 3.7-oz. sprays
Twenty Carats Eau de Parfum	Dana Perfumes	$5	4-oz. bottle; 1½-, 2-, 3-, 4-oz. sprays
Nuance Cologne	Coty	$4.50	4-oz. bottle; 1.8- and 2-oz. sprays

CHAPTER 4

Deodorants, Anti-Perspirants, Feminine Hygiene Preparations, and Douches

In other countries, most people make much less of sweating than Americans do. In Europe and elsewhere, personal odor is simply not a panic item. Before getting into all the products designed to deal with body odors, I should say a little something about sweating in general. Perspiration is one of the body's most ingenious mechanisms. It performs two functions: it cools the body, and it eliminates certain metabolic waste products. Sweat glands are actually intricate little ducts that are present everywhere on the skin. They act as conduits to extract perspiration from adjacent capillaries and deliver it to the surface of the skin, where it can be evaporated into the air. Since evaporation is a cooling process, this helps lower body temperature. Sweat consists mostly of excess water but also contains superfluous salt, ammonia, lactates (chemical byproducts of metabolism), and traces of a host of additional chemicals.

There are two types of perspiration: normal and nervous. Normal perspiration occurs continuously all over the body, and, except after a race in the sun or a game of tennis, it's generally unnoticeable. Nervous perspiration is a neural response to certain brain activities, specifically those related to tension and anxiety. This kind of perspiration occurs in well-demarcated zones such as the palms, soles of the feet, and armpits.

Identical sweat glands deliver both types of perspiration to the skin's surface. The cells at the opposite ends of each duct have opposing electrical charges. This makes the duct work like a sort of miniature electromagnetic pump that literally pulls perspiration out of the body.

At its moment of exit onto the surface of the skin, your perspiration is absolutely odorless. Then why does sweat smell? Because it is immediately set upon by whatever bacteria are resident where it emerges. Bacteria, whose presence on the skin is entirely normal, use the perspiration for their own metabolic processes. I suppose you could say that they "eat" it, except that bacteria don't have mouths and therefore can't "eat" anything in the accepted sense of the word. For organisms that small, you just say they "metabolize." It is the byproducts of this metabolism that can (and usually do) smell bad to us. Each human body is a little universe

DEODORANTS

of its own. Some bodies host bacteria that cause acute odor problems; other bodies just never seem to smell bad due either to scrupulous cleanliness or to comparatively benign surface bacteria.

Modern scientific capitalism has analyzed this situation and come up with two clever approaches to eliminating human body odor. The first, incorporated in the concept of deodorants, is to kill skin bacteria and thereby to avoid the unpleasant-smelling byproducts of bacterial metabolism. The second, as realized in the concept of anti-perspirants, is to temporarily interrupt the natural transportation function of the sweat duct and thereby deprive skin bacteria of perspiration to metabolize. Neither approach is 100% effective, since neither can completely eliminate odor.

Each method does work surprisingly well, but I'm hard pressed to endorse either approach very strongly. For most people, frankly, the best way to avoid body odor is to wash regularly with regular soap. However, there is no evidence that the extra odor protection gained either by killing skin bacteria or by paralyzing the sweat glands is harmful. Skin bacteria replenish themselves; deodorants can't kill them all. And perspiration that is not allowed to flow from a sweat gland due to an application of anti-perspirant will be reabsorbed by the body and excreted elsewhere.

I would not, however, recommend antibacterial deodorants if you already wash with antibacterial deodorant soap. They're redundant and unnecessary unless your odor problem simply won't respond to the soap alone. Similarly, there are times when anti-perspirants are not the answer to excessive perspiration. Certain drugs—cortisone, for instance—actually cause sweating. And some foods—like vinegar, grapefruit, and chocolate—have the same effect. People who suffer from "hyperhydrosis" (medicalese for excessive sweating) may be better off altering their diet on a doctor's advice than slathering their underarms with sweat-inhibiting chemicals.

Here's a medical fact: people who shave their armpits don't smell as much as people who don't. This is because skin bacteria and fresh perspiration are not alone in affecting body odor. Two doctors named H. J. Hurley and W. B. Shelley conducted a number of studies (cited in *The Human Apocrine Sweat Gland in Health and Disease;* Charles C. Thomas, 1960) that show body hair as a major culprit. Hair is a collection site for potentially odor-producing oils and bacteria.

Deodorants work in quite a straightforward way. They simply contain chemicals—the range of which is practically limitless—that kill bacteria. Anti-perspirants, on the other hand, all contain minor variations of something quite different—namely, aluminum salts. The most popular and cheapest salt is aluminum chlorohydrate, but any salt will do, as long as it's derived from aluminum. For some reason, aluminum salts temporarily reverse the electrical charge of the outer end of a sweat duct. This short-circuits the electromagnetic pumping system described above. Anti-perspirants do not work by plugging up pores. They don't have to, because, without opposing charges at opposite ends of the sweat duct, perspiration won't flow to the surface. Fortunately, it won't back up under the skin, either. Instead, it's reabsorbed and the wastes and water contained in it are eventually dissipated through urination, moisture in the breath, and perspiration elsewhere on the body.

Deodorants and anti-perspirants come in many different forms: sticks, sprays, pads, powders, pumps, or what-have-you. Regardless of their form, they all work on either or both of the two principles described above. Occasionally, a product will call itself a "deodorant anti-perspirant." Sometimes this claim has no grounds whatsoever, as the product will be missing either aluminum or an anti-bacterial agent. But sometimes both are present, and the claim is justified. Does that mean the product's guaranteed to work better for you? No, not necessarily. Every human body has its own reaction patterns. "Deodorant anti-perspirants" don't assure superior results. The extra protection they seem to offer is often superfluous.

Many people wonder if it's safe to use deodorants or anti-perspirants every day. The answer is a qualified yes—at least for most people. Now, of course, there is always someone who gets a rash in his or her armpits, but the incidence of reactions like this is not great.

If you do get a rash—which is about the most serious thing that could possibly happen—simply stop using the product and treat the affected area with my all-purpose compress (page 9). The irritation should respond promptly to the compress. You might also wish to write a letter to the manufacturer and describe your experience.

Deodorants

Let's take a look first at bacteria-killing deodorants. The most familiar of these come in spray cans whose propellants will probably all be ecologically safe by the time you read this. My top recommendation goes to RIGHT GUARD DEODORANT, the prototype product in this category. Inexpensive, widely available in drugstores and supermarkets, and effective, it contains a host of polysyllabic antibacterial agents such as benzethonium chloride, SD alcohol 40, and zinc phenolsulfonate. It does not, however, contain any aluminum, since it's not an anti-perspirant. Most other spray deodorants—OLD SPICE DEODORANT or MENNEN PUSH BUTTON DEODORANT, for example—are practically identical to Right Guard save for variations in fragrance.

Helene Curtis Industries has an alternative product that's aimed at people who want to avoid chemical antibacterials. It's called ARM & ARM WITH BAKING SODA DEODORANT, and its effectiveness depends on the mildly antibacterial quality of baking soda. ARM & HAMMER BAKING SODA DEODORANT WITH CORNSTARCH is a similar product. Don't depend on either one of them for heavy odor prevention.

Finally, there are the luxury scented spray deodorants. RIVE GAUCHE GENTLE SPRAY DEODORANT (from Gillette, the same company that makes Right Guard) is typical. The same amount of this product sells for five times the price of Right Guard,

DEODORANTS

but, presumably, it smells the way Yves Saint Laurent himself wants it to smell. It does not, however, offer any additional deodorant protection.

Talcum powder, like baking soda, also has natural antibacterial properties, which is why it's been incorporated into a number of "spray powder" deodorants. I think the best of them is RIGHT GUARD DRY TALC DEODORANT, which also contains aluminum chlorohydrate. Even though it doesn't say so on the label, this is actually an anti-perspirant as well as a deodorant. OLD SPICE DEODORANT POWDER is a more traditional talc deodorant that contains additional antibacterial agents like citric acid, sodium bicarbonate, and salicylic acid—but no aluminum. Medically speaking, sprays containing talc have a lower potential for skin irritation.

Plenty of good spray deodorants also come in the more economical stick form. Among them I recommend MENNEN SPEED STICK, RIGHT GUARD DEODORANT STICK, OLD SPICE STICK DEODORANT, and YARDLEY DEODORANT FOR MEN (which is, of course, equally good for women). The formulas of these products are essentially identical to those in the aerosol spray cans. Finally, for people who don't like either sprays or sticks, there are FIVE DAY ANTIPERSPIRANT DEODORANT PADS. These come in a jar, and each pad is discarded after use. You don't, of course, wait five days between applications; use them as you would use any deodorant. Besides containing antibacterial agents like alcohol and (ready for this one?) methylbenzethonium chloride, Five Day Pads are justified in their anti-perspirant claim since they contain aluminum chlorohydrate.

Anti-Perspirants

The truth is that anti-perspirants are *all the same,* and no one works better than another. All of them contain a minor variation of the same ingredient—namely, aluminum—and no one, as far as I can find, is any more or less safe. Some claim "double" or "extra" strength; my advice is to pay no attention whatsoever to this selling hype. The matter of changing the electrical charges of sweat ducts is a subtle business, and more active ingredient does not necessarily yield greater effectiveness. The same can be said of many substances. For example, Paba, a sunscreen contained in everything from tanning lotions to cosmetics, actually becomes *less* effective in greater concentrations.

Although all anti-perspirant products are equally effective, there is a variable factor—namely, the individual sweat ducts of anti-perspirant users and whether or not these ducts will respond well to application of aluminum salts. Mine do, and my favorite anti-perspirant is RIGHT GUARD ANTI-PERSPIRANT, because it is reasonably priced, widely available, simply concocted, and I happen to like the smell. However, make no mistake, all the products on the following list perform equally well:

> RIGHT GUARD DOUBLE PROTECTION ANTI-PERSPIRANT (which contains a complex of the same aluminum chlorohydrate salt found in the regular Right Guard Anti-Perspirant)

ULTRA BAN 5000 (which comes in Regular, Super Fresh Scent, and Unscented varieties)

ARRID EXTRA DRY ANTIPERSPIRANT SPRAY

ARRID XX EXTRA EXTRA DRY NEW FORMULA ANTIPERSPIRANT SPRAY (with two separate aluminum salts)

DIAL ANTIPERSPIRANTS

DIAL VERY DRY ANTIPERSPIRANT (again, with a double-strength salt of aluminum)

OLD SPICE DOUBLE ACTION ANTI-PERSPIRANT DEODORANT

MENNEN ANTIPERSPIRANT SPRAY DEODORANT (with antibacterial benzethonium chloride as well as aluminum chlorohydrate to temporarily incapacitate your sweat glands)

SUPER DRY SURE (in regular and unscented form)

FRESH NON-STINGING ANTIPERSPIRANT DEODORANT (even though stinging is not really much of a problem with most other deodorants or anti-perspirants)

JEAN NATÉ ANTIPERSPIRANT SPRAY

The following products are now available in nonaerosol pump spray form. Again, they're all practically identical in contents and effectiveness. I give an equal recommendation to:

RIGHT GUARD PUMP SPRAY ANTI-PERSPIRANT (regular and unscented)

ARRID EXTRA DRY ANTIPERSPIRANT PUMP SPRAY (regular and "neutral" scent)

FIVE DAY NON-AEROSOL ANTIPERSPIRANT

MITCHUM NON-AEROSOL ANTIPERSPIRANT (with two separate aluminum salts)

BAN BASIC NON-AEROSOL ANTIPERSPIRANT SPRAY (with the same two aluminum salts contained in Mitchum)

It's almost impossible to find a roll-on that's not an anti-perspirant. So if you like the roll-on form, you'll have to be content with the aluminum-salt approach to inhibiting perspiration flow. The following is a list of recommended roll-on anti-perspirants whose formulas are usually identical to the spray and pump forms of the same brand. All the products on this list perform well—which means that no one is superior to any of the others.

DEODORANTS

    RIGHT GUARD DOUBLE PROTECTION ANTI-PERSPIRANT ROLL-ON

    ULTRA BAN ANTIPERSPIRANT LOTION

    ARRID EXTRA DRY ROLL-ON ANTIPERSPIRANT DEODORANT

    DIAL VERY DRY ROLL-ON ANTIPERSPIRANT

    OLD SPICE ROLL-ON ANTIPERSPIRANT DEODORANT

    BAN QUICK DRY ROLL-ON ANTIPERSPIRANT DEODORANT

    MENNEN BRAKE ANTIPERSPIRANT ROLL-ON

    FIVE DAY ROLL-ON ANTIPERSPIRANT

    TICKLE ROLL-ON ANTIPERSPIRANT

    SURE LONG LASTING ANTIPERSPIRANT ROLL-ON

    JEAN NATÉ ROLL-ON ANTIPERSPIRANT

    MITCHUM ROLL-ON ANTIPERSPIRANT

    BAN ROLL-ON ANTIPERSPIRANT DEODORANT

    YARDLEY ROLL-ON ANTIPERSPIRANT DEODORANT

    ALMAY CHEQ ROLL-ON ANTIPERSPIRANT DEODORANT

    TUSSY ROLL-ON DEODORANT ANTIPERSPIRANT

    REVLON HI & DRI ROLL-ON ANTIPERSPIRANT

Anti-perspirants also come in spray-powder form (for example, RIGHT GUARD POWDER DRY and ARRID EXTRA DRY ANTIPERSPIRANT SPRAY-LIGHT POWDER), in cream form in a jar (as in ODORONO CREAM DEODORANT ANTIPERSPIRANT, MITCHUM CREAM ANTIPERSPIRANT, ARRID CREAM DEODORANT (actually an anti-perspirant very similar to Mitchum), TUSSY CREAM DEODORANT ANTIPERSPIRANT, and FRESH CREAM ANTIPERSPIRANT DEODORANT), and in stick form, too (such as SAFE DRY SOLID ANTIPERSPIRANT and FRESH STICK ANTIPERSPIRANT DEODORANT.) For those who like to spend a little more money for the scent of a good cologne or the name of an exclusive cosmetic house, there are numerous sprays, such as ARAMIS 900 CONCENTRATED ANTIPERSPIRANT SPRAY, PIERRE CARDIN ANTIPERSPIRANT DEODORANT, EAU SAUVAGE SPRAY DEODORANT, GIVENCHY GENTLEMAN DEODORANT ANTI-PERSPIRANT SPRAY, and CHECKMATE DEODORANT ANTIPERSPIRANT, (this last is marketed by Flori Roberts, a house that specializes in cosmetics for black women); and exclusive roll-ons like CLINIQUE ANTIPERSPIRANT DEODORANT ROLL-ON and SCANDIA ULTRA CHEXIT; and even posh spray talcs like KANON MAN'S ANTIPERSPIRANT SPRAY TALC.

    I suppose it is wonderful to have so many choices, even when they don't really differ much. Every one of these products works—and so do the many others with similar aluminum-salt contents that have not been included here for reasons of space. Chosing among them boils down to little more than deciding which smells best, has the most reasonable price, or comes in the nicest-looking package.

Feminine Hygiene Preparations

I join most other physicians in condemning this category of product. First of all, unpleasant vaginal odor is not normal. Its presence is usually a signal that something is wrong. If you're having a problem with odor, it makes more sense to see a doctor than it does to try to camouflage the symptoms with deodorant sprays or inserts.

The word "hygiene" imparts a wholly false scientific aura to these products. They are simply antibacterial deodorants, usually compounded from the same strong chemicals found in underarm products. The vagina, however, is lined with extremely sensitive mucous membrane. Alcohol and benzethonium chloride may not hurt an underarm, but they can—and frequently do—seriously irritate vaginal tissue. Not only is the incidence of irritation high—so is the rate of allergic reaction.

Feminine hygiene sprays are no substitute for plain commonsense cleanliness. To start using them if you have never been troubled by an odor problem is a waste of money and a good way to irritate your vagina. To start using them at the onset of a vaginal odor problem is equally foolhardy; vaginal sprays can do nothing to help the discharge or infection that might be the cause of the odor.

I can't in good conscience recommend one single feminine hygiene product. I would imagine that spray powder formulas like PRISTEEN FEMININE HYGIENE DEODORANT SPRAY POWDER are potentially less irritating than spray mists. I would consider deodorant suppositories like ZONITORS or NORFORMS the worst in terms of their potential for irritation. But, please, if you are having a problem with vaginal odor, *go to a doctor.*

Douches

Douching simply rinses out the vagina. The makers of douching solutions would have us believe that "freshness" is the reason for douching. But, medically speaking, the body is quite able to maintain freshness without douche solutions. The real value of douching lies in its ability to clean out discharges and treat vaginitis.

Vaginitis is a depressingly common inflammation of the vaginal tissues symptomized by an uncomfortable twinge and an itch. The inflammation is usually caused by yeast—an omnipresent small organism (yes, the same thing you bake with)—but any number of bacteria can bring on the same symptoms. Who gets vaginitis? Women who spend too much time in wet bathing suits or in saunas, sportswomen, and women who shower very frequently are prime candidates. Women who take antibiotics while on a course of birth control pills are almost guaranteed to get it.

Douching combats vaginitis by changing the pH (in this case, the level of

DEODORANTS

skin acidity) of the vagina. Douches are all quite acid, and an acid pH inhibits bacteria and yeast. Often, a prophylactic douche is recommended for women on birth control pills who have just started taking antibiotics. This can prevent the otherwise almost inevitable onset of a yeast infection.

One reason for the decline of douching in recent years is that most women don't know the correct way to do it. The key to thorough douching is to keep the outer parts of the vagina closed around the douche nozzle. This prevents the douching solution from running out before it fills and slightly distends the vaginal cavity. This is not in the least painful, and it is necessary in order to reach all parts of the vagina. Position is important, too. One must lie down in a bathtub, knees up and legs slightly spread. When the vagina feels full, the solution should be held within for ten or fifteen seconds, then allowed to gush out quickly. This process should be repeated several times.

There are women who simply enjoy the clean feeling they get from douching. For them, because of the sensitive nature of vaginal tissue, a plain water douche or the use of a bidet is probably best. If you need to alter the pH of your vagina to fight vaginitis, you can do it most easily with a homemade douching solution of one part white vinegar to two parts lukewarm tap water mixed together in a drugstore douche bag. Many of the products below contain citric acid for pH control, but this is in no way superior to plain old vinegar.

Douches come in concentrate form to be mixed with water and used with a douche bag. They also come in disposable bottles complete with disposable nozzles and disposable instructions. It seems like a lot of waste to me, but many women value the convenience.

Of the commercial concentrates, I recommend NEW FRESHNESS first because it is essentially pure filtered vinegar with a wetting agent that encourages efficient cleansing. Other douche concentrates contain a variety of antibacterial and astringent agents that can be irritating if used repeatedly. For example, FEMINIQUE DEODORANT LIQUID CONCENTRATE and DEMURE DEODORANT DOUCHE CONCENTRATE both contain benzethonium chloride; MASSENGILL DOUCHE POWDER contains boric acid and ammonium alum; MASSENGILL LIQUID DOUCHE has SD alcohol 40 and sodium bicarbonate; BETADINE DOUCHE is used mostly in hospitals because of its high iodine content; VAGISEC DOUCHE LIQUID CONCENTRATE has alcohol plus a tongue-twisting assortment of antibacterial agents; and ZONITE LIQUID DOUCHE CONCENTRATE has another strong antibacterial agent called benzalkonium chloride, plus menthol and thymol. Perhaps the most questionable douche compound is in INNER RINSE LIQUID DOUCHE CONCENTRATE, which contains sodium lauryl sulfate (a highly irritating substance), sodium borate, and a high percentage of alcohol. Of course, for each two capfuls of douche concentrate, there is a quart of water that offsets the irritation potential somewhat. But I don't think it's a good idea to apply too much alcohol, alum, boric acid, or strong antibacterials like benzethonium chloride to the sensitive mucous-membrane lining of the vagina. And certainly sodium lauryl sulfate should not be used.

Disposable douches are no gentler than concentrates and a good deal more costly per douche. SUMMER'S EVE, for instance, contains potassium alum as well as more natural citric acid; FEMINIQUE DISPOSABLE DOUCHE has citric acid, too, as well as benzalkonium chloride; MASSENGILL DISPOSABLE DOUCHE has another strong antibacterial called cetylpypidinium chloride, plus SD alcohol 40; and BIDETTE DISPOSABLE DOUCHE has sodium lactate and benzalkonium chloride. Of the disposables, perhaps the gentlest is DISMISS DISPOSABLE DOUCHE. This one contains citric acid, sodium citrate, and a soothing synthetic purcellin oil.

My advice is not to douche regularly with any commercially prepared douche product. If your goal is freshness, douche with plain water. If you're combatting vaginitis, use the one-third white vinegar solution mentioned earlier. Douching occasionally with any of the prepared products listed won't hurt you, but I'll reiterate my recommendation of either New Freshness or Dismiss because of their simple formulas and low potential for irritation.

CHAPTER 5

Creams and Lotions

This chapter is primarily about moisturization and what you can and cannot expect from the various creams, lotions, and ointments on the market. Before getting to specific products, let me tell you about an interesting and very important experiment carried out in 1952 by Dr. Harvey Blank of the University of Miami. The results of his simple experiment cast a penetrating light on the entire cream-lotion-ointment business.

Dr. Blank took hard, calloused pieces of skin and soaked some in oil and others in water for varying lengths of time. Oil, I should note—be it animal, vegetable, mineral, "precious," "exotic," "emollient," "rare," or whatever the label calls it— is the essential ingredient in every moisturizing product. All the hand creams, night creams, moisturizers, wrinkle creams, body lotions, etc., on the market today are basically oily preparations. Well, you'll be interested to know that the calloused skin samples soaked in oil did *not* soften. And the conclusion you can draw is that moisturizers, regardless of the oils they contain, cannot in themselves soften or moisturize the skin.

This is not to say that oil does nothing for dry skin. On the contrary, oily substances do temporarily cement down dry skin flakes. They also lock moisture (water) into the skin by temporarily preventing its evaporation into the air. But no matter how exotic the labels make them sound, oils and "emollients" (a catch-all term for almost anything oily) are simply not skin-softening agents.

Moisturization of any kind is a matter of getting *water* (not oil) into the skin. Once the skin is hydrated, the oil in the moisturizer locks the water in and prevents the symptoms of dehydration—flaking, fissuring, and uncomfortable tautness. This basic principle is the key to moisturizers.

There are many more moisturizing products on the market than are necessary, which complicates matters unduly. In order to market such a proliferation of products, the manufacturers have created a myriad of specific labels. The suggestion in every case is that only a "wrinkle cream" will work on wrinkles, only a "night cream" should be applied at night, only a "body lotion" should be applied to the body, only a "hand lotion" should be put on the hands, etc. Medically speaking, all this diversification is utter nonsense. The products are all so similar that they are literally interchangeable. However, in the absence of this information, the consumer usually makes a purchase on the basis of packaging, scent, or the image that the product has managed to convey via advertising. These all count for something, but none of them bear much on effectiveness.

Let's look at the manufacturers' major categories of creams and lotions and see what really does what. The first five sections that follow deal with creams and lotions whose avowed purpose is strictly moisturization. They include (1) Moisturizers (2) Hand Lotions and Creams (3) Body Lotions, Creams and Ointments (4) Wrinkle Creams, and (5) Night Creams. Three additional sections follow; these list preparations with different purposes; (6) Cold Creams and Cleansers, (7) Bleaching Creams, and (8) Astringents.

Moisturizers

Of course, *you're* the one who has to provide the moisture, which you can do simply by patting the skin with water or by bathing before applying the moisturizer. The oil in every one of these products will then—with varying degrees of effectiveness—lock that moisture in.

I am now going to give you the name of the ultimate hand and body moisturizer. It's a product you already know quite well, and one, I'll bet, that you don't much like to use. Please put your prejudice aside for a moment, because the ultimate moisturizer is pure petroleum jelly, known most widely under the trademark VASELINE.

Now wait just a moment. I know very well that Vaseline is not as cosmetically attractive as a white vanishing cream. But I assure you, without reservation, that Vaseline will prevent the evaporation of moisture out of your skin better than *any other* lotion or cream. You may also think it's too gooey and sticky; that's probably because whenever you used it, you used too much. Unlike many creams and lotions, Vaseline doesn't need to be gobbed onto the skin. It should be applied very sparingly and massaged in well. It takes only a moment to rub it in, and the antievaporation protection it affords is well worth the effort. Throughout this book I'll continue to plug Vaseline in the hopes of chipping away the public's resistance to it. Dermatologically speaking, it's just so much more effective than other moisturizers that it's a shame to let it languish unappreciated.

You can't leave everything up to your moisturizer, though, even if it's Vaseline. If you have dry skin, try to eliminate some of the external causes. You can do this to some extent by humidifying your environment with room humidifiers or simply with shallow tubs of water set out and allowed to evaporate into the air. Plants humidify the air in a room, too; the more plants the better. You can also help dry skin by cutting down on bathing and washing, insofar as is practical. When you do wash, make your bath or shower short, and keep the water a

CREAMS AND LOTIONS

little on the cool side. The hotter the water, the more the pores will open—and the more skin moisture will then evaporate. Sun exposure is also drying, so, if you're really serious about combatting dry skin, cut down on that, too.

But, of course, you can do all these things and still have dry skin. In that case, you should begin moisturizing daily as much as is necessary to ameliorate your own dry-skin problem. There's nothing in any of the following moisturizers that can make you ill. The only thing you must be absolutely certain to do is to *hydrate the skin first.* Get wet, pat dry, and *then* apply the moisturizer.

Although Vaseline is really more than adequate, I should mention another favorite. It's AQUACARE, a unique product that comes in cream or lotion form, and in regular or high-potency formula. Aquacare and the stronger AQUACARE HP both contain urea, a chemical that both attracts and holds moisturizer in the skin. Urea is actually a very ancient moisturizer. If you haven't guessed, it's contained in, er—urine. In fact, as far back as Babylonian times, women were wrapping their legs in urine-soaked towels to avoid dry, cracked skin. The urea in Aquacare (which, incidentally, does *not* come from organic sources) is cosmetically perfectly pleasing. Besides urea, Aquacare contains oily things like petrolatum, glycerine, lanolin, and mineral oil. Regular Aquacare contains 2% urea; Aquacare HP has 10% urea. A competing company puts out urea lotions and creams under the brand name CARMOL. Carmol Ten contains 10% urea, and Carmol Twenty obviously contains twice that. The Carmol products do not contain the same oily moisturizing aids found in Aquacare, so they tend to be absorbed into the skin more quickly. Also good is NUTRAPLUS cream or ointment, both of which contain 10% urea.

Recently, I've been trying a new cream on my patients with dry skin, and the reports I've gotten have been sensational. The product's called SELECTRA CREAM MOISTURIZER, and the active ingredient is—ready for this?—salt! The manufacturers of Selectra apparently are aware of an interesting dermatological tidbit concerning the Dead Sea. Dead Sea water, which has a salt content so high it feels oily to the touch, is exceedingly beneficial to dry skin. The makers of Selectra have composed a formula that is 8% salt (as chemically close as possible to the composition of the Dead Sea) to which they have added traditional oily antievaporation barriers like petrolatum and mineral oil. The result is an excellent product which is, alas, not widely distributed. Better drugstores, if they don't stock it, can order it from Syosset Laboratories, Syosset, New York.

Among the legion of more traditional preparations, I highly recommend NIVEA because of its reasonable price and its availability in drugstores almost everywhere. Nivea comes in cream, lotion, and oil forms and contains familiar oily substances like mineral oil, lanolin, and petrolatum. It's attractively prepared and smells good. The cream form also makes an excellent base to which dry-skinned women can add a few drops of perfume and thereby minimize the drying effect of the alcohol in perfume. In fact, Beiersdorf, Inc., the makers of Nivea, also make a product called EUCERIN, which is essentially Nivea and perfume.

MOISTURIZERS

Many women wonder at what age they should begin using a moisturizer. There is no set age, and some women will *never* need one. However, it's true that, as the human body matures, the production of sebaceous oil on the skin's surface naturally declines. That's why adolescents have so much acne (a condition caused by oil-clogged pores), and it's also why acne tends to decline as people grow older. At least acne is *supposed* to decline as people grow older.

Why, then, is acne the number-one condition that brings adult women to a dermatologist? Because these women are now artificially clogging their pores, not with natural skin oil, but with moisturizers and cosmetics instead. There is so much of this type of acne around that there is even a medical name for it—"acne cosmetica." It is entirely self-induced, by women who erroneously believe they will "damage" their faces by washing with soap. Once that belief takes hold, the face may never be really clean again. The pores become gagged with cold creams and moisturizing oils that seal in the normal byproducts of bacterial metabolism. The bacteria that live on the surface of the skin feed on sebaceous oil, and the byproducts of their metabolism are very irritating. If the face is clean and the pores unclogged, these irritating byproducts can easily be removed during normal washing. But if the face is continually swathed in moisturizing goo, it's like a return to the darkest oiliest days of adolescent breakouts.

When young women who are barely out of adolescence (if that old) start using moisturizers in the misguided belief that they are protecting their skin, the stage is really set for trouble. These women are usually acne prone to begin with. The moisturizer simply makes acne flareups into regular occurrences. If a young face is washed with cream instead of soap, then immediately slathered with a moisturizer, and, finally, caked with makeup, it may just never have a day without disfiguring pimples.

Moisturizers are for dry skin only. If your skin is normal, *don't use them!* I promise, you will not age prematurely without moisturizers, nor will you develop extra wrinkles. In fact, there is no known cosmetic preparation—including the so-called wrinkle creams, which I'll talk about shortly—that can remove, postpone, or prevent wrinkles. Early use of a heavy moisturizing regime that shuns healthy soap and water will not make you look any younger in either the short or long run. It will give you acne, though, to the degree that you are unable to get the oil completely off your skin every day.

It's almost become a rite of passage for young girls to start washing with creams and applying moisturizers and makeup. Believe me, if you don't have to, don't do it. The best protection against acne is to get that face soap-and-water clean every day.

Now, there comes a time when your natural levels of skin oil *do* decline below a desirable level. You'll know that time has arrived when your skin becomes uncomfortably taut, when it feel rough, and looks flaky. Often this only happens on part of your face or body. When it does happen it's time for a moisturizer—assuming, of course, that you have already taken the protective steps mentioned

CREAMS AND LOTIONS

earlier and humidified your environment as much as possible.

For a first moisturizer, particularly on young faces that are just beginning to feel the onset of natural drying, I highly recommend LOVE'S FRESH LEMON FLUFFY MOISTURIZER. If you like lemons (and what American consumer doesn't?) you'll love this stuff. But besides the smell, this product contains SD alcohol 40 and natural lemon oil, two good grease and oil-cutting astringents. It also contains lanolin and isopropyl myristate, two good oily moisture locks. This formula is an attempt to provide moisture protection in a vehicle that is not as acnegenic as traditional super-oily moisturizers. And it actually works quite well.

Let me recommend a few other products that I prefer because they are economical and/or attractive. ALMAY DEEP MIST MOISTURE LOTION has a truly wonderful feel and works very well. LUBRIDERM is nongreasy and very reasonably priced. And, finally, SHEPARD'S CREAM LOTION is a dependable product that's been around for years and years. I like it very much.

As for all other moisturizers on the market, well, they're O. K. if used in moderation on skin that's already been hydrated. The oilier the mixture, the better it'll hold moisture in. The ones with creamy white vanishing formulas, pleasant as they are to use, provide the least effective barrier against evaporation. In fact, they tend to evaporate rather quickly themselves, which is why they are not very useful for really dry skin.

Every moisturizer has some kind of oil-based formula. However—and this is a key point—*no one oil or combination of oils is inherently superior to any other.* To be sure, some products *seem* to work better than others. This is, however, a matter of opinion among the user. Most women who avoid such and such product like the plague do so because it doesn't work for them, personally. This is a matter of individual body chemistry and nothing more. All products—even the ones you hate—have their own loyal following, people who will swear by their effectiveness. Why? Because all products always work on somebody's skin, regardless of how they perform on yours. The products that do the best for the most people are the ones I've highlighted above.

You might find it interesting to see just what oils are contained in other popular moisturizers. What follows is a partial list of these products and their primary oily ingredients.

OILY CONTENT IN MOISTURIZERS

Product	Major Oily Ingredients	Comments
Active Moisturizer (Max Factor)	hydrogenated vegetable oil mineral oil lanolin	a well-priced, well-prepared product and a personal favorite
Aquamarine Moisture Cream	stearic acid isopropyl palmitate	

Continued

MOISTURIZERS

Cont.

Product	Major Oily Ingredients	Comments
Basic Formula for Sensitive Skin (Dorothy Gray)	hydrogenated vegetable oil glycerine lanolin petrolatum	
Body Silk Body Moisturizer (Revlon)	hydrogenated soy glyceride cetyl alcohol propylene glycol	
Cachet Moisturizing Hand and Body Lotion (Prince Matchabelli)	glycerine mineral oil lanolin	
Dermassage Medicated Skin Lotion	mineral oil lanolin urea	contains moisture-attracting and -holding urea
Fabergé Great Skin with NMC—12 Dry Care Moisturizer	mineral oil lanolin propylene glycol Paba	Paba is a sunscreen added presumably to combat moisture loss that might result from sun exposure
Formula 405 Deep Action Moisturizer	mineral oil lanolin	
Houbigant Hand and Body Moisturizer	mineral oil cetyl alcohol lanolin allantoin	
Jergen's Lotion	peanut oil beeswax lanolin	
Jergen's Lotion for Extra Dry Skin	isopropyl palmitate mineral oil	
Keri Cream	mineral oil lanolin	also comes in lotion form
Lanacaine Medicated Dry Skin Lotion	benzocaine	the active ingredient makes dry skin feel better, but it is not an oily moisture-holding substance (and it's also a well-known allergen)

Continued

CREAMS AND LOTIONS

Cont.

Product	Major Oily Ingredients	Comments
L'Oreal Skin Logic	petrolatum mineral oil lanolin urea	
Milk Plus 6 24-Hour Moisturizer (Revlon)	sweet almond oil wheat germ oil sesame oil safflower oil avocado oil castor oil propylene glycol	these vegetable oils are no more effective than mineral oil or petrolatum
Moisture Essence (Max Factor)	propylene glycol glycerol stearate purcellin oil	
Nutraderm Dry Skin Lotion	mineral oil cetyl alcohol	
Oil of Olay	mineral oil castor oil cholesterol	
Pond's Light Moisturizer	glycerine lanolin	
Rain Tree Moisture with NPC	propylene glycol mineral oil lanolin	"NPC" means "natural protein complex," which has no bearing on moisturization
Rich Mer Cocoa Butter Creme	cocoa butter mineral oil triethanolamine	triethanolamine is the basis of Neutrogena soap
Rich Mer Original Vitamin-E-100 Vanishing Cream	same as above with Vitamin E	Vitamin E has not been shown to have any particular moisturizing properties
Rose Milk Skin Care Cream	mineral oil	
Satura Moisture Cream with Vitamin A (Dorothy Gray)	glycerine petrolatum lanolin beeswax mineral oil Vitamin A	Vitamin A has not been shown to be an effective moisture guard

Continued

TWELVE COMMON MOISTURIZER INGREDIENTS

Cont.

Product	Major Oily Ingredients	Comments
Self-Defense Moisturizer (Max Factor)	mineral oil glycerol stearate sesame oil safflower oil	
Silicare Healing and Protective Lotion	propylene glycol allantoin hydrolized animal protein	
Under Makeup Moisture Film (Revlon)	mineral oil propylene glycol urea	
Vaseline Intensive Care	glycerine mineral oil lanolin	very basic, very good, a personal favorite of mine
Wibi Dry Skin Lotion	glycerine	
Yogurt Moisture Concentrate (Max Factor)	yogurt	yogurt has not been shown to be an effective moisture guard

Twelve of the Most Common Moisturizer Ingredients—What They Really Are:

(1) *Hydrogenated vegetable oil* is any normal vegetable oil that has had hydrogen bubbled through it. This process converts the oil to a solid form (like Crisco) so that it can be included in cosmetic products without making them runny. Because vegetable oil is oily, it acts as a barrier to evaporation when spread on the skin.

(2) *Lanolin* is also known as "wool fat" or "wool wax" because it is derived from the oil glands of sheep. It's used in a wide range of cosmetic products—in everything from baby oil to rouge to lipstick to cold cream—because of its ability to absorb and hold water. This capacity, as well as lanolin's naturally oily property, works to substantially improve the emollient (soothing and smoothing) nature of any preparation to which it's added.

(3) *Stearic acid* is a white, waxy, fatty substance that occurs naturally in tallow, butter acids, and a variety of animal fats and oils. It's a moisture lock, meaning it retards evaporation.

(4) *Isopropyl palmitate* usually looks whitish or slightly yellow and is oily/waxy to the touch. It's a natural, organic acid that's derived from the fruits and seeds of palm trees.

(5) *Petrolatum* is also called "petroleum jelly" and is most widely known under the trade name Vaseline. It is a semisolid, nearly insoluble mixture of purified

CREAMS AND LOTIONS

hydrocarbons derived from petroleum. It's the prototype ointment for coating the skin and effectively inhibiting the evaporation of moisture.

(6) *Cetyl alcohol* is a waxy solid substance derived from whale oil. It's a good smoothing emollient, and it helps stabilize oil and water emulsions that would otherwise separate in the container.

(7) *Propylene glycol* is a clear, viscous wetting agent. This substance absorbs and holds moisture and is useful not only on the skin, but also in preventing cosmetic preparations from drying out.

(8) *Urea* is a substance described as "aquaphilic"; by its chemical nature it tends to both attract and hold moisture. Pleasant, odorless urea is derived from uric acid, the same stuff contained (believe it or not) in urine.

(9) *Allantoin* is a synthetically derived (from uric acid), colorless crystal that dissolves in hot water. It's thought to stimulate the growth of new tissue and to aid in the healing of wounds. It feels soothing.

(10) *Glycerol stearates* are white, solid, and waxy. They are emulsifiers, which help stabilize oil and water mixtures and prevent separation of ingredients.

(11) *Purcellin oil* is what makes water roll off a duck. This substance is obtained from the preening glands of water fowl and makes a very good evaporation inhibitor.

(12) *Triethanolamine* is another emulsifier, a substance that aids in the stable combination of otherwise unstable oil and water formulas. It is a colorless solid that also tends to absorb and hold water. When mixed with fatty acids, it forms soap (specifically, Neutrogena soap).

(13) *Hydrolized animal protein* is a coating agent that forms a barrier on any surface to which it's applied. It's something of a blanket term and can refer to any extremely finely ground animal protein.

Incomplete as this list is, it should illustrate just how similar all these moisturizers really are. Less than a half-dozen ingredients reappear continually. In the luxury category, wherein dwell moisturizing products by Elizabeth Arden, Estée Lauder, Diane von Furstenberg, etc., the active ingredients (namely, the oils) are no different and *no more effective* than those listed above. But the price tags on these luxury moisturizers are often way out of line. Top awards for the highest price I've ever seen goes to Orlane, manufacturer of a moisturizer called CREME B-21. Two and a half ounces of B-21 sell for—ready?—$85. Apparently some people actually pay this price, although I know of no possible justification for it.

While we're in the realm of pure baloney, mention must be made of "moisturizers for men." Again, a fallacious suggestion is being made. Men do not need different moisturizers from those used by women. Expensive men's moisturizers by Aramis, Chanel, Clinique, etc., may make a desirable-looking gift package, but there is no medical reason to label them "for men."

A final word before we move on to hand creams: these recommended products notwithstanding (all of them are certainly good), all you really need to properly moisturize skin anywhere on your body is water and a jar of Vaseline.

BODY LOTIONS, CREAMS, OINTMENTS

Hand Lotions and Creams

They look good, they smell nice, but are they really necessary? Let's take a closer look at some of the more popular hand creams and lotions and see if they're really any different from the moisturizers.

My favorite hand product is VASELINE INTENSIVE CARE LOTION EXTRA STRENGTH FOR PROBLEM HANDS. This product contains glycerine (an oily substance that holds water in), petrolatum, and healing zinc oxide (also an excellent sun block and moisture guard). And it's cheap. But don't those active ingredients sound familiar?

I also like JERGEN'S HAND LOTION, which is practically an institution in this country. What's in Jergen's? Peanut oil, beeswax (to give it body), lanolin, SD alcohol 40 (notable for its slishy feel), and synthetic spermaceti (a man-made approximation of whale oil). Again, these ingredients sound mighty familiar.

What contains hydrogenated vegetable oil, petrolatum, and healing allantoin? Answer: JERGEN'S DIRECT AID HAND LOTION. How about a product with glycerine and stearic acid? These are the working ingredients in NEUTROGENA HAND CREAM, in PACQUIN HAND CREAM, and in PACQUIN MEDICATED HAND CREAM (the single "medicated" ingredient being a tongue-twisting antibacterial agent called orthophenylphenol).

All the "hand" products, from the exclusively packaged MOISTURIZING HAND CREAM by Dorothy Gray (which contains propylene glycol, glycerine, stearic acid, cetyl alcohol, lanolin, and mineral oil) to the more democratic JERGEN'S HAND CREAM to "medicated" products, like PACQUIN MEDICATED HAND CREAM are strikingly similar to regular moisturizers. Medically speaking, there is no reason not to use the same moisturizer on your hands that you use on the rest of your body. There is nothing unique to hands that requires a special cream or lotion.

However, for its pleasant scent and silky feel, you may prefer one of these preparations to, say, ordinary Vaseline (which does the job best, despite its cosmetic shortcomings). If you're happy with one of these or with any other hand cream you may be using, stay with it. But remember two things: the drier your hands, the more you'll need products with lots of oil to hold in moisture; and the lighter and more vanishing the cream or lotion, the *less* protection it will provide against dehydration. You can add oil to dry hands until you're blue in the face and it won't accomplish a thing. It's moisture—plain old water—that softens skin. That's what you've got to lock in.

Body Lotions, Creams, Ointments

For better or worse, it is possible in this country to buy something as ordinary as a moisturizer in every conceivable form, scent, color, consistency, and style of package. This is great, as long as the wealth of alternatives doesn't confuse you as to real product effectiveness. In other words, as long as you understand that they all contain approximately the same ingredients and work in the same

CREAMS AND LOTIONS

way, you should be glad you have the option of choosing among so many varieties.

The same situation holds for body lotions, creams, and ointments. They are really no different from hand lotions or moisturizers. The most effective is, once again, the unloved stepchild of the cosmetic industry, VASELINE PURE PETROLEUM JELLY, which is just petrolatum. Vaseline is an ointment, meaning it's oilier and stickier than a cream or lotion. As such, it is much better adapted to sealing moisture into the skin. And it won't leave the skin sticky if you use it sparingly and really rub it in well.

Baby products have been enjoying a recent vogue among users of body creams and lotions. JOHNSON'S BABY CREAM is a good example, and just listen to the active ingredients in it: mineral oil, beeswax, lanolin, paraffin, and glyceryl stearate. Sounds awfully like a hand cream or a moisturizer, right? JOHNSON'S BABY OIL, a favorite of mine, is a good body lotion too, for adults as well as babies. All it is is mineral oil and fragrance. Another popular product is MENNEN BABY MAGIC LOTION. What's in it? Glycerine, cetyl alcohol, and lanolin, plus perhaps a few too many potentially irritating antibacterial chemicals (among them benzalkonium chloride and lapyrium chloride). Other good baby products include JOHNSON'S BABY LOTION (with propylene glycol, beeswax, and cetyl alcohol) and BABY SOFT BODY LOTION (with isopropyl palmitate, propylene glycol, mineral oil, petrolatum, and urea). To judge from the blurb on the package, Baby Soft was never intended for real babies, but rather for those who like to "baby" themselves with "creamy rich" lotions. The ingredients would certainly seem to bolster this claim.

Luxury perfume houses have also gotten into the body lotion act. Everybody from Chanel to Lanvin to Yves Saint Laurent has a heavenly smelling body lotion that matches a cologne. Do they work any better than simple moisturizers? No. Is that a reason not to buy them? Certainly not! By all means go ahead and buy RIVE GAUCHE MOISTURIZING BODY LOTION (about $7 for 8 oz.). After all, it contains mineral oil, lanolin, alcohol, propylene glycol, and urea. Whether or not it's worth that $7 depends on how much you like the scent, the look of the package, and the feel of having something bearing Yves Saint Laurent's name in your bathroom. The same thing can be said of JONTUE BODY SILK, AVIANCE BODY LOTION, EXTREMELY SMOOTHING BODY LOTION and SPECIAL HAND AND BODY LOTION (both by Clinique), CHANEL NO. 19 (and NO. 5) BODY LOTION, ARPEGE MOISTURIZING BODY LOTION, and B 21 CREME FLUIDE FOR BODY AND BUSTE (7 oz. of which is sold by Orlane for the supremely ridiculous price of $45). They're all just minor variations on the same small band of oily ingredients. If you feel the fragrance is worth the surcharge, go ahead and enjoy them. They do, after all, work.

Wrinkle Creams

And what of wrinkle creams? Well, they do make wrinkles look *temporarily* better—first, by smoothing the skin with oil; and, second, by causing a slight irritation. The irritation puffs up the skin just enough to minimize the wrinkle.

WRINKLE CREAMS

No wrinkle preparation can remove wrinkles permanently. It's not possible. Nor can any cosmetic retard the appearance of wrinkles, which result from a combination of exposure to sun and weather plus the natural dehydration that comes with advancing age. You can depend on cosmetic wrinkle creams (or any oil or just plain Vaseline) to make wrinkles look a little better. Just don't think you're making them go away.

The slight irritation that is the hallmark of a wrinkle cream is usually produced by the controversial female hormone estrogen. Granted, the application of estrogen to the surface of the skin is not the same as taking it internally. However, a certain amount of systemic absorption results from topical application. Is this dangerous? It may well be. As you undoubtedly know, a storm of controversy surrounds the use of estrogen in birth control pills and menopausal therapy. It's suspected of being a potential carcinogen, specifically in cases of cancer of the breast and uterus. This suspicion has not yet been positively confirmed, which is why estrogen continues to be widely marketed. Estrogen taken systematically has many positive short-run benefits—to hair, to complexion, to disposition, not to mention as a method of birth control—in addition to its cosmetic effect on wrinkles when applied topically.

But if you are convinced that estrogens are carcinogenic, then you'd better avoid regular use of wrinkle creams. To use them is to inevitably absorb a certain amount into your system.

Dorothy Gray and Helena Rubinstein both make effective wrinkle creams called, respectively, CELLOGEN MOISTURIZING HORMONE CREAM and "PASTEURIZED" FACE CREAM SPECIAL. What they really boil down to is cold cream with estrogen added. Besides creams there are wrinkle sticks, which make spot application easy. Clinique and Etherea make a pair of convenient stick preparations called WRINKLE STICK and WRINKLE GEL STICK. I rate all these products equally effective, with the note that the sticks are perhaps more convenient to carry and use. Let me add that they are all also quite expensive; little 2-oz. jars of the cream cost almost $5, while the sticks cost nearly $7.

Is there an alternative to wrinkle creams? If you go to a dermatologist, he can give you what's called a "mini-peel"—a short application of an irritating chemical—usually trichloracetic acid—to the face. The irritating acid is left on just long enough to provoke a minimal irritation, which in turn provokes a small amount of swelling and "edema," or fluid collection. It's not painful, nor is it terribly expensive. The results last for just a few days, but they really are quite good. The face doesn't look swollen, and the wrinkles are substantially lessened, but a peel is something only a doctor can do.

You can approximate a doctor's mini-peel at home by giving yourself a "rubifactant" mask. Rubifactants are natural irritants; strawberries, pineapple, wintergreen, and lemon juice are all examples of readily available rubifactant ingredients. Look ahead to Chapter 14 for detailed instructions on how to make and apply such a mask.

CREAMS AND LOTIONS

Night Creams

Surprisingly few people seem to be at all aware of the pore-clogging potential of the products we've discussed so far. But the public seems to have a curiously high level of suspicion about night creams. This is ironic, because most night creams (which are marketed specifically for overnight antiwrinkle use) are so similar to ordinary moisturizers that it's hard to tell the difference.

Let's take MOON DROPS DISCOVERY NIGHT CREAM, an attractively formulated product of Revlon, Inc., as an example. The primary ingredients of this cream are sweet almond oil, propylene glycol, beeswax, mineral oil, urea, cetyl alcohol, and hydrolized animal protein. As you can see, the same list could be contained in any moisturizer. So what makes it a "night" cream? Good question.

That question could also be fairly asked of OLAY VITALIZING NIGHT CREAM. The answer is that there is nothing at all about these preparations that makes them particularly suited to overnight application. Again—as you could have guessed—Vaseline applied sparingly after hydration would do just as well.

At least Moon Drops and Olay Vitalizing aren't too terribly overpriced. (Between $4 and $6 for two oz.). But there are people attracted by the luxury night cream blurbs who fork over $20 for less than two ozs. of BORGHESE CREMA DI NOTTE, or (worse) $50 for 1.76 ozs. of Orlane's SUPER HYDRATANTE B 21. Both of these creams are very pleasant, I'm sure, but paying this sort of money for a product whose very designation is dubious seems tantamount to flushing your dollars away. These creams can do nothing—repeat nothing—special for you. They won't even clog pores any better than ordinary moisturizers!

So much for moisturization. We move now to products with quite different purposes, starting with:

Cold Creams and Cleansers

Cold cream may well be the oldest cosmetic preparation in use. First formulated in ancient Greece by the physician Galen, it continues to do what it has been doing for millennia—namely, remove makeup.

Cold creams and related creamy cleansers are *not* substitutes for soap. This is a misconception that has taken unfortunate root in many quarters. It's especially unfortunate in the case of young women who abandon soap in the belief that it is bad for their skins. They wash with cold cream instead—and they get pimples. Why? Because cold cream won't remove acne-causing oil plugs from the pores. It's not strong enough.

Cold cream does do a superlative job of removing the greasy binding materials contained in powders, rouges, lipsticks, foundations, and other makeup. But once you've used cold cream, I recommend that you wash with soap and water to fully remove the emollient residue from both the makeup and the cream. Then,

COLD CREAMS AND CLEANSERS

if you have dry skin, apply a moisturizer to whatever skin areas need it.

Galen's original concoction was made from beeswax, glycerine, and water. It is the evaporation of the water, which starts as soon as the cream touches the face, that gives the skin a sensation of coolness—hence, the name "cold" cream. My top recommendation goes to POND'S COLD CREAM, an excellently priced, widely available, and well-established product that is about as close as you can get to Galen's original formulation. Its simple ingredient list includes (besides water) beeswax, glycerine, mineral oil, and ceresin (a natural mineral derivative very much like beeswax). The instructions, however, do give the impression that "deep cleansing," of the sort that makes soap superfluous, results from use of this product. It's true that older women, whose facial oil glands have become largely inactive, can wash with cold cream alone and not break out. But if you're at all acne prone (and you can be forty and still be acne prone), don't think you're getting your face really clean if you don't use soap.

The practice of using cream instead of soap is being aggressively promoted by the makers of NOXZEMA SKIN CREAM. Ironically, the Noxzema ads all show *young* women abandoning soap in favor of Noxzema, when it is, in fact, this particular segment of the population that should avoid doing such a thing. Noxzema can be too oily for the average young skin. With its clove oil, eucalyptus oil, and camphor, it's a pore-clogger for sure, despite the manufacturer's claim that it *un*clogs pores. Noxzema is great for makeup removal, and even as a smoothing foundation for makeup, but washing with it is no way to keep your skin clean or your pores unclogged. The same thing can be said for NOXZEMA LIQUID SKIN CREAM and NOXZEMA COLD CREAM: great for makeup removal; bad for cleansing.

If you like the products you use to be as simple as possible, let me give you the names of a few more cold creams extremely close to Galen's original formulation. Besides Pond's, there's MOISTURE ENRICHED CREAM CLEANSER (by the Moon Drops Division of Revlon), CLEAN AND CLEAR DEEP MOISTURE FACE CLEANSER (also by Revlon), BASIC FORMULA FOR SENSITIVE SKIN PURE CLEANSER (by Dorothy Gray), MOISTURIZING SALON COLD CREAM (also by Dorothy Gray), and ALMAY HYPOALLERGENIC COLD CREAM (a nice, basic product, even though the "hypoallergenic" claim could be applied to everything on this list).

Some cold creams contain chemical ingredients that bolster somewhat their claims as "cleansers." For instance, Max Factor's GENTLE FOAM CLEANSER contains sodium lauryl sulfate, as does Helena Rubinstein's DEEP CLEANSER. Sodium lauryl sulfate is a strong degreaser. SUPER SKIN DOUBLE ACTION NATURAL CLEANSER FOR OILY SKIN (by Revlon) also has some grounds for calling itself a cleanser. In addition to the usual host of oily cold-cream ingredients, it contains witch hazel, rosewater, and lemon juice, all of which are good astringent degreasers.

In my opinion, some cold creams have too many ingredients, or at least many more than are necessary for simple makeup removal. For example, a product like SUPER SKIN DOUBLE ACTION NATURAL CLEANSER FOR NORMAL OR DRY SKIN (by Revlon) attempts to be a moisturizer as well as a cold cream. It's chockablock with oils

CREAMS AND LOTIONS

(avocado, sweet almond, mint, rosemary, armois, mineral) as well as with the more traditional moisturizing ingredients like propylene glycol and isopropyl myristate. But that's not all; there's also peach juice, urea, and hydrolized animal protein. It's hardly a simple product.

If you're buying cold cream, stick with the simple ones. The cleansers and cleansing cold creams don't really do a good job of cleansing, no matter what the label says. Besides, all those extra ingredients do have some potential for irritation or allergic reaction. The chances are low, to be sure, but I can't see the justification for using a product filled with useless ingredients. That's my main objection to cold creams with, for instance, lecithin (a moisturizer in Max Factor's misleadingly named SUPER CLEAN CLEANSER), or to those with things like wild thyme and sage, which are useless in makeup removal, even though they're contained in REVLON'S NATURAL HERB CLEANSER, or to products with scads of exotic-sounding (and usually acnegenic) oils, such as wheat germ oil, sesame oil, safflower oil, castor oil, and avocado oil—all contained in MILK PLUS 6 CLEANSER by Revlon. Nor can I see any medical justification for paying the luxury prices attached to Clinique's EXTREMELY GENTLE CLEANSING CREAM (which is just a simple cold cream like Pond's) or to Orlane's LACTA-CREME.

Is there any advantage to using liquid cleansers instead of cold creams? No. They are approximately the same as the creams, except that they lack beeswax or any other hardening ingredient. I like Max Factor's MOISTURIZING LIQUID CLEANSER, but only because it's a good, simple product that removes makeup, not because it's inherently superior to cream products. The same is true of ALMAY DEEP MIST CLEANSING LOTION, Dorothy Gray's 2 MINUTE MAGIC LOTION, Etherea's COMPLETE CLEANSING LOTION, and Etherea's OIL CONTROL CLEANSING LOTION.

Don't be misled by labels that make a product sound like the miraculous solution to a skin problem you thought was yours alone. The people who write these labels are very skillful at conveying this sort of impression. Cold cream is cold cream—even when it's in lotion form. And it will *not* get your skin really clean.

Bleaching Creams

This small group of products contains just one major active ingredient: hydroquinone, a chemical that lightens the color of the skin *very gradually*. It's used for evening out dark blotches (usually on faces and hands) that result from normal body chemistry, sun exposure, certain systemic medications, or any combination of these.

Birth control pills, estrogen pills, or merely the state of pregnancy can often result in dark pigmentation of the upper cheeks. This condition is called the "mask of pregnancy," and it's one of the main reasons women—both black and white—buy hydroquinone products. Even when you're not taking any sort of estrogen therapy, it is possible to spontaneously develop dark blotches. It's quite normal, and rarely is it anything to become worried about.

The key to using a bleaching cream is to *always* follow it with a sunscreen (see Chapter 13 for recommendations). If you've developed dark blotches for any reason, *stay out of the sun.* It'll only make your blotches worse. Besides avoiding the sun, be patient. Hydroquinone works, but it takes time—sometimes months.

Bleaching creams often make unnecessary and unfounded claims on their labels. They sometimes suggest that they'll relieve you of everything from blackheads to dry skin. Well, all I can say is that if you have blackheads, use an astringent and squeeze them out, and if you have dry skin, use a moisturizer. Bleaching creams are for gradual spot removal only and shouldn't be depended on for anything else.

I recommend equally ESOTÉRICA (which contains a few soothing oils like lanolin, mineral oil, and allantoin); NUDIT GENTLE SKIN LIGHTENER WITH SUNSCREEN (the inclusion of the sunscreen Paba is laudable, but there's not enough of it to warrant using Nudit without additional sunscreen protection); and ARTRA SKIN TONE CREAM (which is simply hydroquinone.)

Astringents

These products dramatically strip oil and grease from the surface of the skin; they are meant for spot application only. All of them contain alcohol, which causes minor skin irritation, which in turn results in a tightening of the pores. Besides tightening pores and stripping away grease, alcohol has a very drying effect. You may feel refreshed and cooled after using an astringent, but there is a danger of using too much, unduly depleting your skin's natural oil, and thereby inducing uncomfortably dry skin.

The best astringents are plain old witch hazel and humble rubbing alcohol. Both are cheap and available at any pharmacy. The cosmetics industry has, naturally, not been content to leave matters at such a simple pass. So the consumer is faced with a mass of astringent products, each with its own little extra something. Nevertheless, the fact remains that for removing excess oil and tightening the pores, nothing—but nothing—is better than witch hazel or alcohol.

Then why are the cosmetics shelves stacked with "toners," "toning lotions," "pore lotions," "refining lotions," "fresheners," "scruffing lotions," and "exfoliating lotions"? Probably because these labels sound more effective than simple alcohol. Be that as it may, none of the fancy lotions is actually any more effective.

What you're buying when you purchase a toner or pore lotion is a pleasant scent. You can also get a pleasant scent by grating a little lemon peel into rubbing alcohol or putting a few drops of perfume into a bottle of witch hazel. But, to be fair, the commercially prepared astringent products will probably be more attractively packaged and uniquely scented than a home concoction.

My favorite commercially prepared astringent is SEBA-NIL CLEANSER FOR ACNE AND OTHER OILY SKIN CONDITIONS. It comes in lotion and towelette form and consists of alcohol and acetone, two very effective degreasers. I also like SUPER CLEAN UP by

CREAMS AND LOTIONS

the Natural Wonder division of Revlon, whose interesting formula includes witch hazel, lemon juice, rosewater, and lemon oil, plus soothing propylene glycol and allantoin.

The directions on these products correctly note that they are excellent for quick and refreshing cleanups. Some also suggest, with less justification, that they will not cause or contribute to dryness. Toward that end, the formula for Almay's TONING LOTION FOR OILY SKIN contains urea and propylene glycol, Max Factor's SECRET KEY contains talc, and Revlon's TONER FOR NORMAL TO DRY SKIN contains lanolin, isopropyl myristate, and urea. I don't think these or any astringent can possibly be good for dry skin. They all contain too much drying alcohol. Of course if you need an astringent, it's not likely that you *have* dry skin. At least not in those areas where you'd be applying the astringent.

Speaking of application, some of these products also suggest that you apply them to the whole face. This is not at all necessary; apply them to only those areas that are excessively oily. And, although astringents do indeed "fight oiliness," they do so only temporarily. There's nothing in them that will affect either the rate or the location of oil secretion on the face.

Finally, there is the question of astringents "for men," usually called by masculine-sounding names like "scruffing lotions" or "exfoliating lotions." There's absolutely nothing about these products that makes them better suited to men than to women. They all contain the same basic ingredients. Whatever your sex, you can't beat plain alcohol or witch hazel.

CHAPTER 6

Teeth and Breath

Isn't toothpaste the best thing for your teeth? It seems most people think so. Toothpaste, marketed as a fighter of tooth decay, is the second largest-selling cosmetic item (after soap) in the United States. But if you ask any dentist, you'll discover that tooth decay is *not* the number-one tooth problem in the country. That distinction belongs to gum disease, specifically gum recession and the resulting loosening and even loss of the teeth.

The lamentable reality of tooth decay is that its prevention is largely beyond our control. Cavities are primarily a function of the sort of tooth enamel we've inherited. This is a matter of genes, which, as you know, is like Russian roulette. What's more, tooth decay comes in difficult-to-forecast cycles, usually first in adolescence, then at varying intervals in adult life. There is no definite pattern. Every so often, an individual will have a spate of cavities, then a stretch of none at all, then another rush of cavities, etc.

Dental Floss

The best protection against losing one's teeth is regular stimulation of the gums. All the toothpaste in the world won't help a bit. And if your gums bleed easily now, you'd better start massaging them without delay.

Effective stimulation entails three steps: regular flossing; massage with fingers or toothbrush; and regular professional cleaning.

What dental floss does is remove accumulations of "tartar" or "plaque" (two names for the same composite of food debris, enzymes, and bacteria) from the base of the teeth. As tartar builds up, it irritates and pushes the gums back. Brushing, with or without toothpaste, provides only minimal tartar removal. The bristles can't effectively clean between the teeth where the tartar accumulates. If tartar is allowed to build up, the gums may swell, then form germ-catching pockets around the teeth. Finally, the bones and fibers that hold the teeth in the mouth may begin to deteriorate. If nothing is done, the teeth will literally fall out.

TEETH AND BREATH

Flossing is easy, but it's also a pain in the neck. More precisely, it's a pain in the fingers, which all too often get strangled and blue from the floss that's wrapped around them. This is a problem that even good technique doesn't seem to help much.

For those of you who don't already floss, here are simple directions: first, pull about eighteen inches of floss from the spool, hold it at each end between the thumb and index finger and gradually wrap the floss onto each index finger (not too tightly). A one- to two-inch length of floss is then maneuvered between the teeth by using the thumbs and forefingers of both hands. If you can keep tension in the floss with your forefinger, you won't strangle your index fingers.

The best way to get between the teeth (especially if your teeth are closely set) is to floss in front of a mirror. Look at each crevice as you insert the floss; don't try to do it by touch. The floss should go in and out *twice* between each pair of teeth. And while you're in, move the floss back and forth *and* up and down along the sides of the teeth. Remember you're trying to scrape off that gum-irritating plaque, so cover as much of the inner surface as you can. Every few teeth, advance the floss to an unused portion.

When you floss your teeth, you do massage your gums to a certain extent. But you can (and should) do more by rubbing the gums with your toothbrush (back and forth and up and down, but not so hard as to cut yourself, please) or by vigorously rubbing them with the thumb and forefinger. Be certain not to miss any portion. Just a short time per day (thirty seconds) is plenty.

But flossing and toothbrush massage can't do as much as the dentist. Regular professional cleanings every three to six months may seem costly when you're young, but this investment can save a fortune (in tears as well as dollars) if it protects you from "periodontitis" (advanced gum disease) or from the loss of your teeth through gum recession.

The dentist will tell you to floss every day. Should you? Yes, emphatically. But if you do it every other day, you'll still be affording yourself a lot of protection. To do it less than that encourages tooth decay and mouth odor. There is no substitute for dental floss; nothing works nearly as well. If you have difficulty getting it between your teeth, make sure you're getting the "fine"-gauge floss. It's very rare for teeth to be so closely spaced that they can't be cleaned with fine floss and careful maneuvering in front of a mirror.

Dental floss is an ubiquitous and inexpensive drugstore item. It's available "waxed" and "unwaxed" and comes in a number of different gauges, or thicknesses. Waxed floss is easier to slip between the teeth, but my dentist says the unwaxed floss absorbs bacteria better. I believe him.

All brands of dental floss are equally effective—it's a very standard item. There are however, two products I want to bring to your attention. The first is the FLOSS MATE DENTAL FLOSS HANDLE, a small, forked plastic tool that you string with floss and insert into the mouth. This is a dollar item at a drugstore. Alternately, you can try the FLOSPIK, which comes in a package of thirty-two individually wrapped disposable flossing tools prestrung with unwaxed floss. I personally think these tools are the solution (for those who can get the hang of it, anyway) to the strangled-finger problem.

Disclosing Tablets

These products are just becoming popular, and I recommend them very highly. They are an adjunct to flossing that works as follows. Take a tablet, chew it up, and swish it around the mouth. Now stand in front of the bathroom mirror and smile. Every place that plaque has accumulated will be colored bright red. This is supposed to help guide you to the places that need flossing the most.

Johnson & Johnson makes a product called DETECT PLAQUE DISCLOSING TABLETS that you can buy in most drugstores. Rinse the mouth, use the tablets, then floss, then brush. This regimen is for people who are *really* serious about taking care of their teeth.

Toothpaste and Tooth Powder

Volume 33 of the *Journal of the American Dental Association* reports the results of a study carried out by McCauley et al. on the effectiveness of toothpastes and tooth powders. The study involved forty-seven adults who were divided into three groups. Each group brushed twice a day for a period of twelve days with either toothpaste, tooth powder, or plain water. Which group do you think had the cleanest teeth at the end of the test period? If you guessed that any one had cleaner teeth than any other, you were wrong. There was *little* difference in the cleanliness of the teeth of any one group, and the conclusion the experimenters drew was that neither toothpaste nor tooth powder plays a major role in cleaning teeth.

Be that as it may, toothpaste is really very pleasant stuff, and toothpaste manufacturers have some very nifty-tasting foaming formulas. I use toothpaste, myself, but not with any illusion that it is really cleaning or protecting my teeth. It just makes brushing nicer.

The reputation of toothpaste as a tooth cleaner dies hard. What about stains on the teeth? Don't toothpastes scrub them off? Well, for openers, many stains on the enamel of the teeth actually come from *inside* the tooth, meaning there is some systemic cause for them. For example, the public water supply in some places (San Antonio, Texas, is one) contains naturally high levels of "lithium," a chemical doctors use to elevate the moods of psychologically depressed people. Lithium can also cause yellowish-brownish stains to appear on the teeth. Many medicines cause similar reactions. Tetracycline, erythromycin, or any antibiotic that interferes with the normal flora of the mouth can cause such stains. Heavy drinkers get yellowish teeth, too. And these aren't stains you can scrape off.

What about the stains that *can* be scraped off, like those resulting from heavy

TEETH AND BREATH

smoking or excessive coffee drinking? Well, toothpastes can help polish and whiten teeth, but just so much. It's primarily the abrasive action of the brush that cleans the enamel, not the abrasive ingredients in the toothpaste.

Are there any toothpastes or powders with too-strong abrasives that can scratch tooth enamel? The answer to this frequently asked question is an emphatic no. All excessive abrasives have now been eliminated from even the grittiest paste and powder formulas. The ones used today are all essentially variants of chalk, which can't hurt tooth enamel.

What about sticky heavy-smelling "morning mouth"? Doesn't toothpaste get rid of it? Well, it's true that the abrasives and detergents contained in almost all pastes and powders do cut noticeably through the "pellicle," the accumulation found in the mouth upon first waking. But brushing off the pellicle should not be confused with properly safeguarding one's teeth. All those morning mouthfuls of bracing foam simply do not have a significant effect on tooth health or cleanliness. Gum massage and flossing are vastly more important, both to protect your teeth and prevent cavities between them.

What about fluorides? Don't they stop cavities? Well, if you're in the sixth grade or younger, there is indeed some evidence that they do. If you're older than that, chances are fluoride toothpaste may cause you to break out in acne! This is because of the marked similarity in the chemical structure of fluoride and iodine, a noted acnegenic substance thought to trigger the production of excessive skin oil.

Suddenly, from the depths of one's unconscious, comes the sound of an authoritative voice telling us that Crest with stannous fluoride has been "shown to be an effective decay-preventive dentifrice that can be of significant value when used in a conscientiously applied program of oral hygiene and regular professional care." Thus spake the Council on Dental Therapeutics—American Dental Association. In point of fact, they can say the same thing about almost any toothpaste, because the point of this seeming endorsement is not to sell Crest, but rather to get you to brush regularly and go to the dentist. That's what the last phrase means; "conscientiously applied" brushing, and "regular professional care" at the dentist keep inaccessible areas of the teeth clean. The mention of Crest (or any brand) is almost incidental.

When you pay for a tube of toothpaste or a can of tooth powder, you're getting a pleasant taste (by far the biggest factor influencing consumer choice of these products), plus a collection of mildly helpful but not necessary chemicals. Principal among these are the following: fluorides (which combat cavities only in young children); abrasives (to help cut through the pellicle); surfactants (which break down the surface tension of the pellicle); and humectants (to attract and hold moisture).

Toothpaste and tooth powder do help, but only a little. I recommend that you buy either the best tasting or the cheapest brand and not be hornswoggled by extravagant claims or quotes. AIM, CLOSE-UP, PEPSODENT, LISTERINE, MACLEANS, CREST,

COLGATE, GLEEM, and ULTRA-BRITE are all the same—as far as medical effectiveness goes.

As for the slightly grittier preparations—like PEARL DROPS TOOTH POLISH, DR. LYON'S TOOTH POWDER (my preference), COLGATE TOOTH POWDER, etc.—they're just as safe for the enamel as regular pastes. I actually prefer grittier formulas because they scrub off the pellicle faster (but not any better) than pastes or plain water. They're also cheaper, although all these products are rather cheap to start with.

If you have sensitive teeth and wince with pain every time they come in contact with cold, heat, sweets, sour tastes, or plain bites of food, I recommend SENSODYNE, which contains strontium chloride to help form a protective barrier on the teeth. THERMODENT, with sodium bicarbonate, sodium chloride, potassium sulfate, and a solution of formaldehyde, does the same thing. Both preparations mix their active desensitizing ingredients with a regular-flavored dentifrice. In my opinion, they are both equally effective.

What about exotic specialty toothpastes? Is clay and sea salt (contained in BARTH'S SEA GEL) the real secret to whiter teeth? No, at least not any more than the chalk and saccharin in Crest. How about that black tooth powder called MONKEY BRAND imported from India? Assuming you can get it, it won't do anything special for your teeth. About the only thing that can be said for these products—as well as for others containing fennel flavoring (the hallmark of TOM'S NATURAL TOOTHPASTE), limestone and Vitamin A (as in DOLOMITE), or red dye to heighten the contrast between teeth and gums (which is how EMAIL DIAMANT, a French import, works)—is that they make an amusing change of pace.

Mouthwash

Here's a good chance to save some money. All you have to do is *not* buy mouthwash. It is a product that does not affect the smell of your breath for any significant period of time. It's just like a room freshener—the effect is fleeting and the product does nothing whatever to get at the cause of the odor.

All that can be said for mouthwashes is that they are simple concoctions; they are innocuous but not useful. Essentially, they're all variations on four major ingredients: water; alcohol; flavor (usually saccharin); and artificial color. Besides doing nothing for bad breath, mouthwashes do nothing to relieve throat pain or fight colds in any way—and the government has at last gotten the manufacturers to stop claiming that they do.

Let's look for a moment at the causes of bad breath:

(1) First and foremost is lack of adequate brushing and flossing. The bacteria that normally live in the mouth metabolize food particles caught in the teeth, and in the process they produce bad odors. Keep the teeth clean, and this won't happen. These same bacteria are at work in cavities, or under dentures, but, again, if you keep your mouth clean and go to the dentist regularly, you'll keep bacteria problems to a minimum. The alcohol in mouthwash is a natural antibacte-

TEETH AND BREATH

rial agent, but it only temporarily depletes their number. Almost any mouth will return to premouthwash condition within two hours of use. And sometimes continual use of mouthwash will actually encourage stronger odor-producing strains of bacteria.

(2) Sometimes certain substances—they differ from individual to individual—interact unpleasantly with mouth bacteria. It may be onions, or coffee, or cigarettes, but whatever it is, the best way to deal with it is by brushing and flossing.

(3) Although 90% of breath odor stems from poorly cleaned teeth, a substantial 10% comes from the lungs. Garlic provides a good example of how this works. Garlic is a substance that once in the bloodstream is easily exchanged with the air in the lungs. Brush as you will, you won't dispel garlic breath, because it's coming from your lungs. Other substances, for example, the tranquilizers stellazine and thorazine, amphetamines, and the antibiotic tetracycline, often have the same effect.

(4) Much odor-producing bacteria, sloughed-off skin cells, and food particles are naturally cleared from the mouth by swallowing. Dryness of the mouth, which inhibits this normal odor-clearing process, will therefore also tend to encourage bad breath. Cold remedies that dry the nose typically have the same effect on the mouth, which means that Allerest, Contac, Benedril, and any other antihistamine remedy will usually encourage unpleasant breath. The unnaturally dry climate in an airplane does the same thing; perpetual mouth breathers suffer similarly.

Children usually have sweet breath, but the older one gets the heavier the breath becomes. Everybody's breath is most pungent upon awakening, particularly if one has a gum disease or breathes through the mouth. The biggest cause of morning breath is the putrefaction of skin cells shed during the night. The next biggest cause stems from mouth bacteria that have been at work overnight on food debris or in cavities. Much of this odor is dispelled quickly by swallowing and talking. This, plus a good brushing, is enough to freshen most mouths.

Mouthwashes can't clean the teeth, nor can they affect lung odors in any way. Their antibacterial properties are temporary and even a potential hazard if they kill benign mouth bacteria and encourage the substitution of strong odor-producing varieties. Because mouthwash is only temporarily effective, there are people who gargle the stuff all day long. If they use a product that contains boric acid (for example, Listerine) they may well get a dose of boric acid poisoning. An early symptom of this condition is accelerated hair loss. It's extremely difficult to diagnose and, fortunately, the damage is temporary. But it's also the last straw, as far as I'm concerned, on the subject of mouthwash.

I must be blunt; you're foolish to use mouthwash regularly. It's a waste of money and a potential (if remote) hazard. Using mouthwash to get rid of bad breath is like painting your face to get rid of acne, so I can't in good conscience recommend any mouthwash products. They all taste good, which is really the basis on which they are sold. But they're baloney; don't buy them.

Toothbrushes

I don't think I've ever bought a toothbrush in my life—dentists have been handing them to me free since I was a child. I was amazed, therefore, to find that there is such a wide range of toothbrushes available, in colors and bristle types to please everyone.

As far as clean, healthy teeth and fresh breath go, the act of brushing is far more important than the type of brush used. Dentists seem evenly divided on the advisability of hard or soft bristles, and the collective professional mind seems to swerve back and forth on the issue every few years. Perhaps to accommodate this indecisiveness, most toothbrush manufacturers make "hard," "soft," and (just to be safe) "medium" bristle models. I have yet to run across a toothbrush that wasn't well made, so I think your purchase decision (assuming that you, too, don't get your brushes free) must rest on the type of bristle you prefer.

My first choice is ORAL-B, which is for people who like soft bristles. That's the only kind they make, and they point out on their label that "a toothbrush does not have to hurt to work." Oral-B comes in three-row models for children and four-row models for adults, is very soft, and costs around a dollar.

PY-CO-PAY SOFTEX is similarly soft, a little cheaper, and comes with that little rubber tip at the end of the handle. They call it the "Pycotip" and make much of its ability to stimulate the gums between the teeth. You can do this much better with dental floss. Just to cover the field, the same company makes the slightly harder regular model PY-CO-PAY (with nylon bristles) and the harder yet PY-CO-PAY NATURAL BRISTLE (with natural, unbleached bristles). There is no medical advantage to natural bristles; they're for people with a prejudice against nylon. All Py-co-pay brushes come equipped with the Pycotip.

LACTONA is another soft-bristle brush with a rubber tip similar to the Pycotip. The same company also manufactures the LACTONA NATURAL, whose natural bristles come in medium, hard, or extra hard varieties. The cost is again around a dollar.

Other less expensive brushes that come with either hard or soft bristles include the TEK PROFESSIONAL, the ANGLE SYNTON (supposedly sculptured for more effective cleaning), and Squibb's 1600 STRAIGHT HANDLE TOOTHBRUSH (at under 50¢, the least expensive of our survey samples).

Two specialty brushes bear note. The SENSODYNE is a gentle-bristle brush specially made for sensitive teeth. It won't hurt orthodontic bands or artificial dental materials, either. Finally, there's the LAPIDENT, a curious toothbrush that contains its own toothpaste chamber. Fill it up, follow the directions, and the brush automatically dispenses paste onto its own bristles. Hmmmmmmm.

Denture Cleaners

The best way to keep dentures clean is to employ the same method people use to keep real teeth clean—namely, brushing. I recommend an extra-hard-bristle

TEETH AND BREATH

denture brush, such as the COLGATE DENTURE DELUXE or the WERNET DENTURE BRUSH. Use either regular toothpaste or, if you prefer, try DENTU-CREME TOOTHPASTE FOR CLEANING FALSE TEETH. Actually, any type of toothpaste will work equally well—don't expect too much.

Brushing dentures is, however, far more thorough than dropping them into a cup of chemicalized water overnight. As a nation, we seem to love things that plop and fizz—especially if they turn colors, as denture effervescents do. Well, all those green and blue fizzy cleaners like POLIDENT, EFFERDENT, KLEENITE, etc., have no more cleaning power than two tablespoons of salt in a cup of lukewarm water. Certainly they are no substitute for the cleaning action of a thorough brushing.

My advice: to really clean and deodorize dentures, brush, don't soak.

Denture Adhesives

The trouble with denture adhesives is that most of them are made with "space-age" plastics that can cause allergic reactions. At least enough of them do to make natural formulations preferable.

Just as moisturizers themselves don't provide moisture, but rather lock water into the skin, so denture adhesives themselves don't hold dentures in place, but rather create an airtight seal and a vacuum that do the job. Which product works best is a highly individual matter. The answer depends on a host of variables—the shape of your mouth, the age of your dentures, the chemical nature of your saliva, the condition of your gums, etc.

There are three approaches to holding false teeth in the mouth: powders; creams; and cushions. Powders are sprinkled on clean, damp dentures, which are then pressed into the mouth and allowed a few minutes to set. Creams are applied in strips to clean, dry dentures and inserted the same way. Some products claim to hold dentures firmly in place for up to four days, but I doubt this. Besides, dentures really have to come out for cleaning every evening. As for cushions, they are only temporary measures to mitigate the discomfort of poorly fitting false teeth. They are to be used only until you can get to the dentist.

I like FASTEETH DENTURE ADHESIVE POWDER and EASO DENTURE ADHESIVE POWDER best, because they contain benign natural ingredients and no plastics. The adhesive in each is karaya gum mixed with sodium borate, and it performs well. It's true that most people will not have any noticeable adverse reaction to the plastic adhesives found in nearly every other adhesive product. If you like a powder form and don't care about plastics, you can try WERNET'S DENTURE ADHESIVE POWDER (also available in a "super" formula for "hard to hold" dentures), COREGA, POLIDENT, LACTONA, or EXTRA STRENGTH EFFERGRIP. These are all good adhesives with long-standing reputations.

Some of the same companies—for example, Wernet and Effergrip—make cream versions of their powder formulas for people who prefer that type of adhesive.

DENTURE ADHESIVES

Other equally effective cream preparations include ORAFIX (which also comes in a "special" formula for older dentures), POLI-GRIP (also available in "super" formula), FIXODENT, BRACE, CONFIDENT, and CUSHION GRIP.

Cushions again are only temporary measures. But they are enormously helpful when your dentures are killing you and there's no way to get to the dentist for days or weeks. EASO DENTURE CUSHIONS come in packets specially cut to fit both upper and lower plates. They're probably the easiest cushions to use and are available in regular and heavy gauges.

SNUG DENTURE CUSHIONS and PLASTI-LINER TEMPORARY DENTURE RELINERS are much more complicated affairs, requiring you to do your own trimming and fitting. Instead of a dozen disposable cushions for daily use (as with Easo), Snug has but two pads (one for the upper plate and one for the lower) and Plasti-Liner but one. I would resort to either of these products only if your fit problem won't respond to Easo cushions. And remember: cushions are *temporary* measures only.

CHAPTER 7

Makeup

I've changed my mind about makeup. I used to be thoroughly against it, having time and again in my practice seen evidence of its one big drawback. That is the horribly widespread incidence of "acne cosmetica"—acne breakouts in adult women due to makeup-clogged pores.

However, after much thought and study, it's now my feeling that acne cosmetica is due not so much to the makeup itself as it is to incorrect and/or excessive application. What's more, despite the hazards and hassles of acne cosmetica, it's a dermatological fact that makeup protects skin from pollution and sun exposure. My own preference for a natural, un-madeup look notwithstanding, I have to say that older women who've used makeup all their lives have smoother and better preserved skin than women who haven't. And that's a persuasive reason for using makeup.

This isn't to say, however, that makeup is a necessity. It's not, and if you don't use it every day the extra wrinkles you may pick up certainly won't impair your health or estrange your loved ones. The impact of makeup on one's self-image is really what's important—far more important than its incidental capacity to enhance skin preservation.

Many people seem to think makeup is dangerous. Well, it's not. It *rarely* causes allergic reactions, be it an ethereally packaged hypoallergenic tube from a swank department store or a 59-cent item from the local five and dime. Every manufacturer tests his product exhaustively before loosing it on the public. People seem very cynical about business these days, but take my word for it: all cosmetic preparations are thoroughly tested. They aren't even marketed unless human test volunteers show an incidence of allergic sensitization that is less than 1 in 10,000. Don't forget that there is no such thing as a substance to which *nobody* is allergic. Ten thousand to one is good odds.

People always want to know why cosmetics cost so much. Well, without doubt the big factor is packaging and image projection. I suppose there is some logic to making a product that looks so glamorous on the pages of *Vogue* cost more than 59¢. Buying a page of advertising in *Vogue* isn't cheap, either. But it's also true that the ingredients in cosmetics vary minimally from product to product. And many products are not even manufactured by the houses whose labels they bear. Rather, the preparation is subcontracted to major producers, who do the concocting for many different cosmetics houses.

Inexpensive makeup is—at least medically speaking—absolutely the equal of costly makeup. The only substantial difference is color. Generally speaking, the exclusive houses are very good at coming up with shades that are both fashionable and rich looking. The dime store usually doesn't have the same knack. But with makeup, it's quite possible to hit a Brand X dime-store item that just happens to have a terrific color. Be it lipstick, nail polish, cheek gloss, or whatever, if the color is good, by all means buy it.

Speaking of color, another question frequently heard bears on the safety of makeup dyes. Again, preproduction testing establishes a reasonable measure of safety for all cosmetics ingredients. However, it does seem that there's always some dye or other suddenly being revealed as a potential carcinogen. The chances of absorbing a dangerous amount of dye into your system by using makeup are very low. Years ago, makeups contained toxic lead- and mercury-based pigments, but no more. In the United States there hasn't been a case of systemic toxicity related to makeup for many, many years.

Whatever you do, don't become muddle headed on the next subject—"purity." Products that tout themselves as "pure" and "organic" are no more safe than those that contain man-made chemicals. In fact, no cosmetic is really 100% organic. Chemical preservatives are a necessity without which cosmetics would rapidly rot. It's also just as easy to become irritated or allergic to natural ingredients as it is to chemical ones. "Natural" is not inherently better, it's just more expensive.

Although I am not opposed to the use of makeup, I do think it should be applied sparingly. Unfortunately, there are no established directions for applying makeup. What some women use as foundation, others use as a touchup; colors and creams that some women cake on daily others don't use at all. I think makeup lessons are a great idea. If you can resist the strong pressure to purchase cosmetics, I would recommend that you go to one of the big salons like Elizabeth Arden, pay the $20 or $30, and take a lesson. If you don't live close to a famous salon, there's probably a major department store somewhere near you that can offer the same service. But perhaps the best idea is to get a copy of famous makeup artist Way Bandy's fine book *Designing Your Face* (Random House, 1960). Bandy is a famous pro, and the book is well worth the price. It's amazing what you can learn about application—even if you've been using makeup for years.

How about the most efficient methods of makeup removal? I have very definite advice on this subject, which you'll find in Chapter 1: Keeping Face and Body Clean. Then, preparing the face for makeup application is a critical matter only if you have dry skin. For instance, using a facial steamer or stepping fresh from a hot shower will leave your pores wide open and your face well hydrated. Immediately splashing on cool water will tighten the pores and retard moisture

MAKEUP

loss. Additional application of a moisturizer and/or makeup will further retard moisture loss by forming a barrier coat on the surface of the skin to prevent evaporation. Sealing moisture in like this is good for dry skin. It's not necessary if your skin is normal or oily.

The balance of this chapter is divided into eleven sections:

(1) Foundation Makeups
(2) Concealers
(3) Face Powders
(4) Cheek Glosses and Blushers
(5) Lipsticks and Glosses
(6) Eyeshadows and Eye Colors (for application to the upper lid)
(7) Mascaras
(8) Eye Liners
(9) Eye Pencils
(10) Eyelash Adhesives
(11) Face Blotters

Foundation Makeups

The purpose of a foundation makeup is fourfold: it smoothes and fills in skin imperfections; it adds color to the complexion; it protects skin from the environment; and it provides a base (here's where the word "foundation" comes in) for additional makeup. This is not to say all foundations must be followed by more makeup. It's purely a matter of whether or not you want to add more color to your face.

Foundations come in cream and liquid forms, neither of which is inherently superior. Face powders, discussed below, can and often do perform the job of foundation makeups just as well as any cream or liquid. All three forms have about the same potential to clog your pores—if you use too much of them and/or don't wash your face at night with soap and water.

Let me tell you the latest medical thinking on water-based vs. oil-based cosmetics. Water-based products (all of which, incidentally, contain at least some oily ingredients) are lighter, and therefore it would seem logical that they are less likely to clog pores. Remember that clogged pores are step one in the development of acne breakouts. However, in actual practice it's the amount of makeup, not whether it's oil or water based, that most influences the incidence of breakouts. If you're young and/or acne prone, it won't make much difference which makeup you use as long as you apply it sparingly.

If you're in the midst of active acne breakouts, be especially sparing in the application of any makeup. A better idea would be to use a disaster cream (see recommendations in Chapter 10: Acne Preparations). Putting makeup on over breakouts only delays their healing.

FOUNDATION MAKEUPS

Clear preparations are the lightest makeup available and are typically about 75% water. Foundations containing pigments are usually 50% water, with the balance made up of coloring agents plus oils similar to those in the clear products. Besides oils, water, and pigments, makeups all contain "emulsifiers" to mix the oil and water, "humectants" to attract and hold skin moisture, and "barrier agents" like zinc oxide, titanium, or sunscreens, to protect against the environment.

Cake makeup, despite the unfortunate "pancake" image, is probably better for oily/acne-prone skin since it covers exceptionally well and tends to sop up oil.

What follows is a list of recommended sheer makeups, about the lightest you can get. They're for normal to oily faces that don't need a lot of cover.

NATURAL WONDER OIL-FREE SHEER MAKEUP (by Revlon; highly recommended; also comes in a "medicated" form that contains an astringent called parachloro-meta-xylenol)

BASIC MAKEUP OIL-BLOTTING FORMULA (by Charles Revson; highly recommended; in ten shades)

FRESH COVER LIQUID MAKEUP (by Helena Rubinstein)

FRESH & LOVELY OIL CONTROL MAKEUP (a very reasonably priced Maybelline product that comes in nine different shades)

ULTRA LUCENT OIL-FREE PURE MOISTURE FLUID MAKEUP (by Max Factor; in eleven shades)

ALL DAY OIL CONTROL MAKEUP (by Cover Girl; in five shades)

SHEER MAKEUP (by Cover Girl)

OIL FREE GEL MAKEUP (by Love; in five shades)

You'll note that most of these products come in more than one skin shade. You can also have your pharmacist custom tint makeup (or any skin product you buy) by means of the Dermik Labs Color Blender. Most good drugstores offer this service, wherein the pharmacist consults with you over a color chart and helps you choose a coloring agent that will make your makeup blend exactly with your natural skin tones.

Let me note here that the Flori Roberts Company of Neptune, New Jersey, has for years been specializing in makeup for black women. Their MELANIN MAKEUP BASE and MELANA SOUFFLÉ are both nicely formulated covering products. But the price, I think, is high. Especially when you can have a less expensive product custom tinted with the Dermik Blender. Don't be shy; go ahead and ask your pharmacist about "color blending." Remember though, this is a custom service, not the sort you'll find at a big discount drug mart.

If you have oily or very oily skin and are intent on using makeup despite the risk of acne, then I strongly recommend Max Factor's PAN CAKE MAKEUP. This

MAKEUP

product is inexpensive and covers very well. If applied sparingly (you use a sponge) it will not look cakey. And remarkably enough, despite the "rich oils" touted on the label, Pan Cake actually seems to absorb skin oil and provide a measure of protection against breakouts. I like it too because it's a one-step product. Since it comes in colors, you don't have to put anything else on top of it.

As skin grows older, it produces less natural oils. This means your face can gradually tolerate heavier makeups. Acne breakouts connected with makeup do continue, however, to plague women right into their forties. Even if you're not a kid anymore, always be careful not to use too much. The following products contain more oils than those listed above, and they also tend to cover imperfections more effectively. They're slightly heavier, but not much.

FACE QUENCHER (by Chapstick; highly recommended; in six shades)

HONEST MAKEUP (by Bonne Bell, an excellent manufacturer of effective, reasonably priced cosmetics)

FRESH & LOVELY MOISTURE WHIP (by Maybelline; priced right and available in six shades)

GLOWING FINISH ALL IN ONE MAKEUP (by Coty)

MOISTURE WEAR LIQUID MOISTURE MAKEUP (by Cover Girl; in six shades)

CREAM MOISTURE MAKEUP (by Cover Girl; similar to the last recommendation but in cream form)

CLEAN MAKEUP (by Cover Girl; in five shades)

PORTRAIT LIQUID MAKEUP (by Yardley of London)

HI-FI FLUID MAKEUP (by Max Factor)

CREME-PUFF MAKEUP (by Max Factor)

SUPER CLEAR MAKEUP WITH LECITHIN (a nice product by Max Factor, even though the lecithin probably doesn't do anything for the skin)

BABE COUNTRY FACE COLORS (by Fabergé; good colors but expensive)

TRULY NATURAL FACE COLOR (by Frances Denney; again, quite expensive)

B 21 MAKEUP (a good product from Orlane, but the price—$25 for a little over an ounce—is ridiculous)

FLAME GLO MAKEUP MOISTURE (by Flame Glo; cheap and effective)

PAN STIK MAKEUP (by Max Factor; in easy-to-apply stick form)

CONCEALERS

Recently there's been a fashion for "translucent" makeup. These foundations—used either singly or in combination with glosses or blushes for the cheeks—are clear enough to see right through. The idea is to give the face a glowing, dewy look, but application isn't always easy. Too many women put on too much and wind up looking strangely shiny. With a light touch on a clear complexion, the effect is very attractive. The following list contains brand names of recommended translucent-look makeups.

> TRANSPARENT COLOR GLAZE (by Etherea)
>
> TRANSLUCENT CREME MAKEUP FOR NORMAL/DRY SKIN (by Etherea)
>
> TRANSLUCENT CREME MAKEUP FOR OILY SKIN (by Etherea)
>
> C. H. REVSON EXTRAORDINARY FACE MAKEUP (by Charles Revson division of Revlon)
>
> WHOLESOME MAKEUP ALL-DAY FACE TINT (by Charles of the Ritz)
>
> FLUITONE MAKEUP FOUNDATION FOR NORMAL AND OILY SKIN (by Scandia)
>
> BASIC MAKEUP FOR NORMAL/DRY SKIN (by Etherea)

If your skin is mature and/or dry and you feel you need lots of coverage, you can use a heavier foundation makeup. CLINIQUE'S CONTINUOUS COVERAGE and Scandia's MAKE-A-TINT MAKEUP FOUNDATION are both recommended examples of fairly heavy, oil-laden preparations. These and others like them *really* cover; don't use them unless you need to.

Time and again, I've cautioned you to apply foundation makeup sparingly. Now here's how: dot the makeup onto the skin with the fingertips in the following sequence: cheeks first; then chin; finally, the forehead (the throat is optional). With the fingers, blend the makeup up and out from the nose. The sequence applies whether or not you intend to add additional color. In the case of pancake makeup, use the sponge that comes with the makeup following the same sequence and stroke pattern.

Concealers

Of course, regular foundation makeup is really a "concealer." But there are specially designated "concealer" products that do what mere makeup cannot. These opaque preparations—usually marketed in lipstick-type dispensers—paint over imperfections. The cosmetic companies describe this as "lighting out" shadows in areas such as the forehead, under the eyes, and around the nose and mouth. Concealers also obliterate visible evidence of tiny lines, blemishes, and skin discolorations. They do all this when applied as a first step under makeup. If you develop a good technique, you can also use a concealer on top of makeup

MAKEUP

to slim the nose, accent the cheeks, build up the chin—or at least give that illusion.

Typical stick concealers contain oils (like mineral or lanolin), talc, a heavy covering agent (like zinc oxide or titanium dioxide), and beeswax (to make them stiff enough for the lipstick dispenser). My top three choices among the many available are Max Factor's ERACE (also available in a waterproof formula with a mascara-type dispenser), Almay's COVER UP STICK, and Revlon's HIGHLIGHT WHITE VANISHING STICK. These products cost less than three dollars and are available in drug and department stores almost everywhere. Clinique's CONCEALING STICK and Etherea's WRINKLE GELSTICK are also good products, but they cost more than twice as much as the suggestions above and don't do the job any better. The lipstick-type tubes are designed to be dabbed on lightly, then blended with the fingers.

For women who prefer cream-form concealers, I recomend Almay's UNDER EYE COVER CREME (whose use is certainly not limited to just the eye area) and Scandia's RETOUCH COVER-UP CREAM (expensive, but very effective).

Even though it's not marketed specifically as a concealer, I highly recommend Max Factor's PAN STIK MAKEUP, because it combines the jobs of makeup and concealer in one simple step. The stick dispenser by its very nature discourages excessive application, too.

Two final points must be made about concealers. The first is that plain Vaseline when applied alone or under makeup will also minimize tiny lines and wrinkles. The second is that concealers, while as safe as any other cosmetic, are exceptionally pore clogging. Don't use them on acne-prone areas, and certainly not over active breakouts. You can hide those with the disaster creams described in Chapter 10.

Face Powders

Face powders these days are skillfully prepared, very attractively packaged, and have a shelf life that's almost indefinite. Essentially, they're all made of talc, variously processed and tinted. They can be used as a foundation, or they can be applied over a cream or liquid foundation makeup; and they're great for end-of-the-day touchups on top of existing makeup. How (or whether or not) you use them depends entirely on how much coverage you want.

All powders tend to reduce shine and give an attractively smooth glowing look. The danger, as ever, is overapplication. Powder won't hurt you, but it can look cakey and crack if applied too liberally and can clog pores as well as any cream or liquid makeup. Personally, I think a good powder that's close to your natural skin tone makes an excellent color-evener and can stand on its own as a one-step makeup. To use powder on top of makeup is to move inexorably away from a natural look.

Face powders come in loose and pressed form, the former with a puff, the latter with a pad, sponge, or brush-type applicator. I like ALMAY in both pressed and loose form because of its quality, consistency, and reasonable price. The same goes for NATURAL WONDER OIL FREE PRESSED POWDER by Revlon. INTEGRA and CLINIQUE (both loose and pressed) are also very good but cost more than twice as much as the Almay and Revlon products.

Many powders come in different colors. I think Max Factor's ULTRA LUCENT WHIPPED CREME PRESSED POWDER ("whipped" simply indicates the presence of additional air) gives you effective coloring at a reasonable price. Charles of the Ritz's REVENESCENCE POWDERGLOW, and Clinique's SOFTLY SHEER (both available in loose and pressed form) do an equally effective job for twice Max Factor's price. Expensive powders are *no better* than less expensive powders. But again, there is the matter of good color. Sometimes to get exactly the shade you want requires paying a higher price.

I particularly like CLINIQUE TRANSPARENT BUFFER because of its handy brush and compact form and its nice polishing properties. I don't care much for Flori Roberts's MELANIN FACE POWDER which, despite a handy shaker bottle, is overpriced, apparently solely because it's aimed at black women. Other powders are just as effective on black skin tones and it's not necessary to pay the premium price just for the Flori Roberts label.

Cheek Glosses and Blushers

Creme blushers, powder blushers, and cheek gels are all modern updates of one of the oldest types of makeup in the world—rouge. These substances can be applied either under makeup, over makeup as a finishing touch, or all by themselves. The makers of blushers and glosses print all sorts of puffy label claims about their special moisturizing ingredients and uniquely natural look. I wouldn't expect any therapeutic effect from these products. Nor would I expect them to appear too natural. But they're quite safe and easy to use, and they do add color.

It's my opinion that too many women use too much cheek gloss. A little color is one thing, but aggressively crimson cheeks look anything but natural. Ironic, isn't it, since all the cheek color makers repeatedly chant the praises of looking "natural."

Most cheek products are applied with the fingers, although manufacturers are consistently coming up with "improved" applicators. The color should be initially applied high on the cheekbone at a point approximately below the outer corner of the eye. It should then be smoothed upwards and outwards toward the hairline at the temple. The area to be colored should in no event extend beyond an imaginary boundary line straight down the cheek from the center of the eye.

Once again, price differentials reflect nothing as far as medical purity, hypoallergenicity, or effectiveness. High prices do correlate to the images of fancy cosmetics houses. The following cheek-color products offer the best value for the price (usually $2 to $3).

MAKEUP

    NATURAL WONDER KEEP BLUSHING (by Revlon)

    NATURE'S BLUSH (by Coty)

    TRUE BLUSH (by Bonne Bell)

    CHEEK-GLO ROUGE (by Cheek Glo; creme or powder)

At a slightly higher price ($3 to $4) are the following:

    FRESH COVER BLUSHING CREAM (by Helena Rubinstein)

    WHIP CREME BLUSH (by Almay)

    GLOWING FINISH CREMEPOWDER BLUSH (by Coty)

    BABE COUNTRY CHEEK COLORS (by Fabergé)

    ULTRALUCENT WHIPPED CREME BLUSH (by Max Factor)

Clinique, Etherea, Scandia, and the Polly Bergen Company, among a host of others, make enough cheek blushers, gels, and powders to fill anybody's dressing table. They usually cost twice as much as the ones listed above, for which you get only the name and perhaps a color not available elsewhere. The same may be said of Flori Roberts's LIQUID GLO. Why this cheek color for black women should cost twice as much as Revlon's Natural Wonder Keep Blushing is a mystery to me. There's certainly no medical basis for it.

Lipsticks and Glosses

Lipsticks are rather simple formulations concocted of an oil (upon which lipstick makers love to lavish extravagant descriptions), plus pigment and wax (to make it rigid enough to be molded into a stick). The only difference between standard lipstick and little pots of lip gloss is the presence of more wax in the stick and more oil in the gloss.

Lipsticks really do help protect lips from drying environments. But, wait a moment, if you're really suffering from dry lips, you should be using oily barrier agents like Chapstick, Aquaphore or Vaseline. Lipsticks and glosses are also barriers against evaporation, and, as such, they will help hold moisture in lips, but only to a limited degree. Don't be confused by "moisturizing" or "emollient" ingredient claims. The primary reason for oily substances is to allow lip products to spread evenly and stick to the lips. Remember, oils don't moisturize, they only hold moisture in. Manufacturers may say what they will about moisturization, but don't let these claims be the basis for your purchase.

I think the purchase of lipstick or lip gloss should be based purely on low price and desirable color. Expensive sticks and glosses offer absolutely nothing either medically or cosmetically superior to the cheaper brands. There is a whole range of luxury lip-color products, and, for the life of me, I can't find any justification for their high prices. What's more, these are precisely the type of cosmetics that are regularly subcontracted out for manufacture. There are anonymous factories at this very moment parceling out lots of the same day's production to be packaged elsewhere and sold for wildly different prices.

Medical problems arising from the use of lipstick or gloss are rare; the mouth is one of the least likely parts of the body to experience allergic type problems. Many people do suffer from herpes (cold sores), and lipsticks can actually help this condition, as they shield the lips from the sun, which is thought to be connected with herpes eruptions.

So, I would say that if you like colored lips, do wear all the lipstick you want. If you have a problem with dry lips, lipstick and gloss will help a bit, but your real treatment should be Chapstick, Aquaphore, or Vaseline. And, when you're buying lip colors, you might just as well shop for the less expensive ones. The following is a list of my favorite reasonably priced (about $1.75 to $2.50) lipsticks, all of which come in many shades.

MAXI-MOIST LIPSTICK (by Max Factor; highly recommended)

LIP COLOR (by Maybelline; highly recommended)

FROST FORMULA 2 (by Revlon; highly recommended)

LIP SOFTENERS (by Cover Girl)

LOVESTICKS (by Love)

SILKSTICKS (by Coty)

LIPSTICK (by Natural Wonder)

ULTRALUCENT WHIPPED CREME LIPSTICK (by Max Factor)

FABERGÉ LIPSTICK (by Fabergé)

CREAM CARE AND FROST CARE LIPSTICKS (by Helena Rubinstein)

BABE COUNTRY LIP COLORS (by Fabergé)

CREME TINT LIPSTICKS (by Almay)

CREME LIP ACCENTS (by L'Oreal)

The following list encompasses an exceptionally wide range of interesting colors. However, these all cost twice as much as they should ($4 to $6).

REVENESCENCE LIPSTICK (by Charles of the Ritz)

HALSTON LIPSTICK (by Halston)

CHARLIE EXTRA EXTRA SHINE LIPSTICK (by Revlon)

RE-NUTRIV RICH RICH LIPSTICK (by Estée Lauder)

LIPSTICK (by Christian Dior)

MAKEUP

       PRINCIPESSA LIPSTICK (by Princess Marcella Borghese)

       RE-MOISTURIZING LIPSTICK (by Clinique)

       DIFFERENT LIPSTICK (by Clinique)

       SPECIAL FORMULA LIPSTICK (by Etherea)

       SHINING LIPSTICK (by Etherea)

What is said of lipsticks can also be said of lip glosses; there is no medical or cosmetic basis for the high prices attached to the luxury segment of the market. All lip glosses are, for all practical purposes, the same.

Because of their higher oil content, lip glosses give a more shiny and moist look to the lips. Unless packaged with an applicator, they're applied with the tip of the finger. Color is applied first to the center of the top lip, moving out to each side, then to the lower lip. Applying a colorless lip gloss over a colored one gives an even higher shine.

Here is my list of recommended, reasonably priced ($2 to $2.50) lip glosses.

       AUTOMATIC SUPER SHINY LIP COLOR (by Maybelline; highly recommended)

       CREME SHINE LIP COLOR (by Max Factor; highly recommended)

       POT O' GLOSS (by Yardley of London; highly recommended)

       SHINE MAKER (by Cover Girl)

       COLOR 'N GLEAM (by Almay)

       GLOSS CARE (by Helena Rubinstein)

       NATURAL WONDER SHINY SHINY LIP GLOSS (by Revlon)

       LUSH LIPS (by Flame Glo)

       NATURAL LUSTRE LIP GLOSS (by Aziza)

Finally, let me note that Clinique, Chanel, Etherea, and a score of other luxury cosmetics houses also make lip glosses that are absolutely the equal of those listed above. The trouble is that their prices are not equal—they're twice as high. But O. K., if they've got the color you want, and paying $4 for a little pot of gloss bothers you not, go ahead and buy.

Eyeshadows and Eye Colors (for application to the upper lid)

Do you know the most common hazard connected to the use of eye cosmetics? It's not allergic reactions to the eye-makeup products, nor is it skin irritation. It is, surprisingly enough, allergic reaction to nail polish! You see, many women do their nails and eyes in the same sitting, and it's very common to flick the

EYESHADOWS AND EYE COLORS

lashes with nails that aren't completely dry. Result: allergic redness or irritated swelling of the eyelid. People assume it's a result of eye cosmetics, but no, it's most often a result of exposing tender eye tissue to nail enamels.

Eye cosmetics are more rigorously tested and stringently regulated by the government than any other cosmetic product. The days when they contained questionable ingredients are long past. I know consumers tend to resist the type of statement I'm about to make, but facts are facts—eye shadows and colors are very benign concoctions.

According to every manufacturer, today's eye shadows and colors won't crease or settle in lid lines; won't streak, separate, or smear; will stay on all day; are waterproof (and tearproof, too, although it seems to me you'd have to hang upside down and cry to find out for sure); won't fade; will protect tender eye skin with "rich," "gentle," "soothing," and "encapsulated" emollients; are easy to apply; come in many many "terrific," "shimmering" shades; and make your eyes look "exciting," "glamorous," "interesting," "impressive," "expressive," and "bigger."

Take a little oil, a little water, a bit of pigment, plus an optional dash of pure aluminum for iridescence, put it in a compact with a brush applicator, and, presto, you've got eyeshadow. Apply it to the lid area bounded by the lashes and the brow and suddenly your eyes look "interesting," "impressive," "expressive," and maybe "bigger."

All eyeshadows are quite safe to use. Even if you get them in your eyes, a quick flush with either Visine or a solution of salt water will put you back to rights in a flash.

The following is a list of my favorite eyeshadows. Why are they my favorites? Because they're sensibly priced ($2 or so) and come in plenty of different colors.

AUTOMATIC CREAM-ON SHADOW, ULTRA FROST, ULTRA VELVET, PEARLY ULTRA FROST (by Maybelline)

ONE STROKE EYE COLOR (by Cover Girl)

WATERPROOF EYE SHADOW, CREME-ON EYE SHADOW, WHIPPED CREME ENRICHED EYE SHADOW, MAXI-RICH SHADOW (by Max Factor)

NATURAL WONDER (by Revlon)

COLOR RICH EYE SHADOW (by Almay)

Of all other shadows, I will simply state again that if the color pleases you and the price is agreeable, too, it's safe to assume the product, whatever it is, is as safe and effective as any on the above list. Let me mention in passing that I personally like the unusual muted earth shades available in Fabergé's BABE EYE SHADOW line, and in Bonne Bell's COLORADO COLORS SPRING EYESHADOWS. Since many women use two different eye-shadow colors, you might also like to know about

MAKEUP

Etherea's MOISTURIZING EYE SHADOW DUAL PLAN, a single compact containing two harmonizing high-fashion tones. Finally, if fingers and brush-type applicators aren't for you, then maybe you'd like a soft pencil-type eye shadow. In that case, Revlon's NATURAL WONDER SHINING EYECRAYON PENCIL and Max Factor's HI-FI EYE SHADOW STICK might be just the ticket.

Mascaras

Mascara is basically a waxy, pigmented coating that makes lashes look thicker. I love the label claims on mascara products—they know no shame! Whatever you do, don't read just one label and think, Aha! this product does everything! Because they *all* "lengthen," "thicken," "fluffen" (!), "separate," "curl," and "color." And they're all smear resistant, tearproof, and long lasting and, properly applied, none of them will cause clumps. Ever.

Like all eye products, mascara is rigidly tested to conform to perhaps the only really strict set of government guidelines in the cosmetics industry. Whether the label says it or not, every mascara is about as dermatologist-tested and hypoallergenic as it can be. Years ago they used coal-tar dyes in mascara products, and many irritations resulted. Today the pigments are all benign. About the only irritation I've ever seen in connection with mascara stemmed from (believe it or not) women diluting it with saliva. This actually can increase the chance of infection.

There are three basic types of mascara applicators: brushes (in varying sizes); wands; and combs. I personally think the little combs separate, spread the color, and curl best, but, of course, I don't wear mascara. Here is a list of reasonably priced and highly recommended comb applicator mascaras.

LASH MAKER AUTOMATIC COMB ON MASCARA (by Max Factor)

LOOK NATURAL COMB-ON MASCARA (by Maybelline)

SUPER LASH MAKER COMB ON, BRUSH ON, ROLL ON MASCARA (by Max Factor)

This last product combines all three methods of application in one unique applicator. Considering Max Factor's fine reputation as a manufacturer, plus the reasonable price of the product and the versatility of the applicator, I give it my top recommendation.

Brush-type mascaras abound, and among them I would recommend the following, primarily on the basis of their reasonable price.

BRUSH TIP MASCARA, MAXI-LASH MASCARA, LASH FULL MASCARA (by Max Factor)

FLATTERLASH MASCARA (by Fabergé)

COVER GIRL LONG 'N LUSH MASCARA (by Noxell)

LONG LASH MASCARA (by Helena Rubinstein)

AZIZA MASCARA WITH CONDITIONER (by Prince Matchabelli)

A word about mascara with "conditioner." Aziza makes much of this, but, frankly, I've rarely heard of anything so silly as conditioning your eyelashes. Fortunately, Aziza is a good mascara at a good price—despite the somewhat frenzied promotional concept.

Finally, if you like a wand-type applicator, I recommend Max Factor's MASCARA WAND, which is effective and reasonably priced.

I cannot in any event see spending $4, $5 or $6 for any mascara. To my mind, this effectively rules out the mascaras by Clinique, Etherea, Lancôme, Scandia, etc. They're fine products, but the high prices seem unjustified.

Mascara, in case you don't already know, must be applied in a few coats to achieve the desired effect. It is most important to wait at least a minute between coats to avoid clumping. And whether you use brush, comb, or wand, stroke upwards on the upper lash and downwards on the lower lash.

Eye Liners

By painting a thick line on the outside of either (or both) lids, as close to the lashes as possible, one can make the eyes appear more wide open. Sometimes this effect is very attractive; sometimes it's superfluous; and sometimes it's plain ridiculous. Many women look better *without* accenting the eyes so strongly, but, of course, this is an entirely subjective matter.

Eye liners—be they pencil, powder, or liquid—are quite safe, even for the sensitive skin at the rim of the eyelid. Eye liners are also waterproof, tearproof, and often soap-and-water-proof too. (Fortunately, cold cream always removes 'em.)

My favorite eye-liner values are Helena Rubinstein's MINUTE LIQUID LINER and Max Factor's LINEMAKERS STAY ON LINER and HI-FI FLUID EYE-LINER. These all have little brush-type applicators and cost less than three dollars. You can, of course, spend twice as much and get the same thing from Clinique or Etherea.

Two luxury products that offer a little something extra for their prices do come to mind. Clinique's BASIC EYE EMPHASIZER is a sheer powder that comes in a subtle tone of gray (only one color) and is used as a liner, eye shadow, and brow definer. It's nice, and very low key. Scandia's INTEGRA EYE SHADOLINER is a sleek compact containing brush and sponge applicators to shadow and line eyes in five different shades. Again, nice and low key, and it does offer something not available in every eye-liner product.

MAKEUP

Eye Pencils

These products have a dual function. Their primary use is to fill in sparse areas of the eyebrows with short, feathery strokes to give a more dramatic look. They are also used as eye liners, but, frankly, I think the liners mentioned above might be a little safer to use around the eye than a pencil.

The most basic eye pencil—also the best buy—is Maybelline's BROW PENCIL and companion LINER PENCIL. At a half a dollar apiece, they can't be beat for value. But keeping them sharp isn't always so convenient. There are two ways to approach sharpening: one is to buy a product that comes with a sharpener; the other is to buy an automatic pencil. Almay makes a good product, packaged with two sharpeners, for under $2.50; it's called SKETCHSTIX CREME SHADOW PENCIL, and I recommend it highly. For another half-dollar, you can buy their EYEBROW PENCIL WITH BUILT-IN SHARPENER. Perhaps a better deal is Helena Rubinstein's automatic MINUTE FINELINE PENCIL for about $2. Equally good are automatics from Almay (FINELINE EYE PENCIL) and Max Factor (FINE LINE AUTOMATIC EYE PENCIL).

Regardless of form, all eye pencils are benign concoctions of various pigments plus waxy ingredients to make them stiff enough to draw on flesh. Like all eye products described so far, they are quite safe—and almost identical to one another.

Eyelash Adhesives

You may very well have an allergic reaction to an eyelash adhesive. Lots of people do. That's why using mascara is vastly preferable to false eyelashes.

The trouble with eyelash adhesives is the adhesive plasticizers. These things just aren't good for human skin. To be sure, the manufacturers do everything possible to test for incidence of irritation and/or allergic reaction. And if you do use false lashes, you can take some comfort in the knowledge that once the adhesive sets, the allergic danger passes. But, again, if you possibly can, stick with mascara. I think this is an important point, and for that reason I cannot really recommend any specific adhesive products.

Face Blotters

Here is a useful little product that does just exactly what it claims to—and no more. Face blotters are for oily-skinned women who occasionally need to blot up excess oil but don't want to disturb their makeup. The blotters themselves are small, pure linen squares packaged in "purse-pacs" of several hundred. They cost about a penny apiece or less and contain literally nothing that could possibly hurt you. Two good brands of face blotters are SHINE OFFS PURE LINEN FACIAL BLOTTERS (by Celebrity, Inc.) and ANDREA FRESH-UPS (by Andrea Raab Corp.), both available in drugstores.

CHAPTER 8

Fingernail Products

In a way, nail products are cosmetics at their best, because they can really improve your physical appearance. But they're also cosmetics at their silliest—because they unblushingly make extravagant and groundless health claims.

To begin with, nail products frequently make much of their supposed ability to strengthen the nails. Well, it's absolutely true that if you paint any hard coating onto the nail you'll strengthen it; that's the obvious result of painting a hard coating on anything. But, no matter what it says on the label, there is *no* known ingredient that will make the nails themselves either become or begin to grow out harder or more resistant to splitting, cracking, and so forth.

What makes nails strong and split resistant? Well, I'll tell you right away that drinking protein or gelatin has nothing to do with it. The basis for this old wives' tale is the fact that fingernails themselves are protein substances. However nails grow from the skin adjacent to them, specifically from the "nail fold" (the area below the cuticle at the base of the nail) and the "nail bed" (the area beneath the nail itself). If the skin here is unhealthy, the nails will be, too. And drinking protein has nothing to do with the health of this skin. Nails also reflect the overall health of the body; many systemic problems can disfigure them. Finally, the healthiest and best-looking nails are invariably found on hands that stay clear of irritating chemicals, traumatic blows, and frequent immersion in water.

Nail products are wonderful at covering damaged nails, but to improve the nail itself you must do more than paint it over. It helps to understand that fingernails are quite dead, a characteristic they share with hair. But for water content and a stray mineral or two, hair and nails are practically identical protein structures. No matter what you put on your head, you can't make hair grow. The same thing goes for nails. The most you can really do to maintain your nails in their healthiest possible condition—and this is the medical truth, surprising as it may be—is to maintain the nail folds from which they grow and the nail beds on which they rest.

When the skin of the nail fold becomes inflamed, you've got trouble. Eczema,

FINGERNAIL PRODUCTS

psoriasis, lichen planus, or any inflammation that affects the skin anywhere can affect the skin of the nail fold. This can and usually does lead to pitted, cracked, and deformed nails. Besides, fungal, bacterial, or yeast infections (from, for instance, constantly washing dishes or doing anything that keeps your hands wet all day) can irritate the nail fold and cause future nail growth to suffer.

Nail beds, by contrast, are more prone to allergic reactions—for example, to fake-nail adhesives or nail hardeners. Allergic reaction in the nail bed, depending on severity, can ultimately result in the nail falling completely off the finger.

Fingernails mirror overall physical health, too. If you are iron deficient, your nails may become spooned; if you lack sufficient calcium, they may become alarmingly dry and brittle; they may even turn green if your metabolism is awry; blue if you suffer from chronic heart disease; or pale and yellowy if you have diabetes.

So, it is a combination of environment (meaning the way you use your hands every day) and overall physical health that determines the health and appearance of the fingernails. You can't put anything on them to make those problems go away.

Nail products are not only good coverups, but are all essentially hypoallergenic—even the ones that don't say so. Allergy problems (except to certain products I'll discuss below) are infrequent, and, once any of these products dries, the chance of allergic reaction is drastically cut. That's why "quick-drying" formulas are always preferable.

I've divided popular nail products into the following seven categories:

(1) Nail Polishes
(2) Nail Polish Removers
(3) Artificial Nails
(4) Nail and Cuticle Treatments
(5) Nail Fortifiers (for use before and after enamel application)
(6) Cuticle Removers
(7) Nail-Tip Whiteners

Nail Polishes

All nail polishes are equal—except for the desirability of certain colors. The very best salons frequently use the cheapest nail polishes with their manicures, so you might as well use them, too. If you can find a good color in a cheapie "Brand X" polish from the local five and dime, you're ahead of the game.

Nail polish is just paint, so please don't be swayed by extravagant label copy. I know it says the stuff "protects your nails against splitting, chipping or peeling" but so would refrigerator enamel. Whether an expensive polish contains "conditioners," is "dermatologist tested," has "natural emollients," or weird additives

NAIL POLISHES

like nylon, it won't—it can't—do any more for your nails than an inexpensive product like MAYBELLINE NAIL COLOR (my favorite, incidentally, in twenty-four different shades).

You should buy nail polish with two criteria in mind: attractive color and quick-drying formula for protection against allergic reaction. No nail polish is likely to really improve the existing condition of fingernails, either. Polishes all contain tough chemicals—polymers, plasticizers, solvents, resins, etc. Tossing in a few emollients or oils to "condition" is laughable. They're simply overpowered by the main ingredients.

Can nail polishes hurt you? I don't really think so, but nobody knows for sure. The F. D. A. has recently received complaints from women who experience nausea after applying nail enamel. Is this from inhaling the fumes? Or does it stem from absorption of ingredients into the system? No one knows for sure. There's some talk at present about the potential carcinogenicity of nail-enamel dyes. But if there's a connection between cancer and nail polish, nobody's established it yet. One thing's for sure, though, and that is that nail polish will *not* improve the condition (call it "health" if you must) of fingernails.

So many inexpensive nail polishes come in wide color ranges that it's hard to find a good reason to buy luxury nail polish at all. The following is a list of recommended polishes that, a silly claim or two notwithstanding, are all reasonably priced.

MAYBELLINE NAIL COLOR (by Maybelline; highly recommended)

NAIL GLAZE (by Fabergé)

CREME NAIL ACCENTS (by L'Oreal)

COVER GIRL "NAIL SLICKS" (by Noxell)

ULTRALUCENT WHIPPED CREME NAIL ENAMEL, and MAXI-WEAR NAIL GUARD (by Max Factor)

ALOISE NAIL POLISH (by Aloise)

CLEAR COVER SLICKER NAIL POLISH (by Yardley of London)

CREME NAIL ENAMEL (by Almay)

HARD AS NAILS WITH NYLON (by Sally Hansen)

STRONG & ICY (by Helena Rubinstein)

As for Estée Lauder, Clinique, Chanel, Charles of the Ritz, Etherea, and the ever-expensive Orlane (a little bottle of whose "6 CARATS" NAIL ENAMEL costs $4.50), well, what can I say? The colors are lovely, the packaging superb, but is there anything in these polishes that will either make them look better on or improve the condition of your nails? No, nothing whatsoever.

FINGERNAIL PRODUCTS

Nail Polish Removers

There is just nothing about nail-polish remover that could possibly be construed as good for your nails. That doesn't stop the manufacturers of these products from broadly suggesting that they will "condition" your cuticles (an amusing concept wholly without medical basis) or "moisturize" your nails.

The "exclusive" moisturizer that purports to do these things usually turns out to be a dash of lanolin—which is totally overwhelmed by the other ingredients. The most common polish-remover ingredient is acetone, a toxic chemical that efficiently wipes enamel off the nail. If the product contains no acetone, then it's probably based on benzine. Whether or not it contains any additional oils or perfumes, polish remover by its very nature is going to strip away skin oils and hasten the evaporation of moisture from porous fingernails. Now, if you immediately apply a new coat of polish, you'll probably seal existing moisture into the nails before it has a chance to evaporate; you may never even notice that your polish remover had any drying effect at all. If you use polish remover frequently but don't reapply polish promptly, you'll face the same sort of dry-nail problems faced by people whose daily tasks expose their hands to strong chemicals or water.

Let me interject here that human beings aren't fragile creatures. If you get stains on your nails from using nail polish, that's just because nails are porous. The stains won't affect the condition of your nails. And if you dry out your nails with polish remover—and it really takes a lot of polish remover to do this—it's very easy to put the damage to rights by hydrating the nails at home. Here is a simple hydrating regimen: dip the fingers into lukewarm water for two minutes, pat dry, and massage a *small* amount of Vaseline into the fingertips. If you don't care for Vaseline, use Aquacare or your favorite skin moisturizer. What you're doing is sealing the moisture into your cuticles, nails, and surrounding skin. You don't need any special nail conditioner or moisturizer to do that.

My favorite product is CUTEX OILY NAIL POLISH REMOVER—not because it claims to condition the cuticles (which is nonsense), but because of its simple acetone-based formula and reasonable price. Cosmetics houses with fancy names charge five and six times as much for polish removers that are in no way superior. Also reasonably priced are FABERGÉ NAIL GLAZE REMOVER and MAX FACTOR NAIL POLISH REMOVER. If you find an inexpensive dime-store brand, by all means use it.

There's no point listing all the overpriced nail-polish removers on the market. Suffice it to say that you should beware of claims like: "won't strip nails of natural oils" (they *all* do); "hypoallergenic" (they *all* are); "with moisturizers and conditioners" (baloney); "for the life your nails have to lead" (nails are dead); etc. Some moderately priced products also make silly claims, but you should forgive them if they at least don't overcharge. Remember: the way to combat dry, flaky nails is to hydrate and seal in the moisture.

For truly lazy people there are also nail-polish remover pads. These products are uneconomical and do not remove nail polish any better than the liquids. It goes without saying that they also are incapable of "conditioning" nails or cuticles. I suppose under some circumstances they might prove convenient. They come in individually wrapped packets, each one of which holds a pad supposedly capable of doing all ten nails. My advice: buy a bottle of Cutex.

Artificial Nails

Throughout this book I've been reiterating how safe most cosmetics really are. Well, here is one of the exceptions. Artificial nails are a dangerous product, and I actively discourage their use.

The problem is they're made of highly allergenic plastics and come with similarly allergenic adhesives. It's a pity, really, since they're so cleverly packaged and conceived. With good technique you could give yourself a fantastic-looking set of phony nails whose authenticity no one would ever doubt. But, if you are among the many who experience an allergic reaction in the nail bed, your whole nail would fall out.

Fake nails—either those that are glued on or those that are built onto the nails by means of successive painted coats—are equally bad, to my mind. Again, it's true that many women do use them without problems, but the prospect of a nail falling out is truly horrendous, sometimes almost crippling. And the nail that grows back will invariably be deformed or somehow not quite right. Fake nails are not worth the risk, and I cannot possibly make any product recommendations.

Nail and Cuticle Treatments

Products in this category promise to either "condition" nails and cuticles or "strengthen" nails prone to splitting and cracking. Let's take a closer look at what's really going on.

Just as oil alone cannot moisturize the skin, it cannot moisturize nails or cuticles, either. As a matter of fact, "special" nail and cuticle oils bear an amazing resemblance to regular hand creams and moisturizers. They are simply cosmetically attractive creams containing various oily substances plus perfume. These oils are effective only to the degree that they seal in moisture.

People who regularly use nail polish and nail-polish remover are prime candidates for dried-out nails and cuticles. Should they then rush out and buy nail conditioners or cuticle oil? Well, in my opinion there is no point in buying a special nail or cuticle product. The best way to keep nails and cuticles from looking dried out and/or cracked is, once again, by hydrating the fingertips by immersing them in water (two minutes is *plenty*), then massaging in your favorite hand cream, body lotion, or moisturizer, or (my favorite because it seals in water best) Vaseline.

FINGERNAIL PRODUCTS

There is no lack of products that claim to be "expressly created for dry and brittle nails" or that "strengthen nails by preventing dryness" or that contain impressive-sounding ingredients like "natural collagen," "protein," "nylon," and so on. Don't be fooled. None of them does a single thing for the nail fold from which the nail grows. In combination with hydration, *any* oily nail or cuticle treatment will help seal in moisture, but probably not as well as Vaseline. And probably no better than your favorite hand cream or moisturizer, either.

If your nails do suffer from chronic dryness, brittleness, and splitting, it makes much more sense to eliminate the most common causes of this condition. If your hands are in water too frequently each day, wear rubber gloves. If in the course of a day you must constantly touch drying substances, chemicals, or other materials, go to the drugstore and get "fingercots." These look like little rubber caps that pull on over the finger tips. Perhaps you're washing your hands too often or using too much drying soap; if so, cut back. Or you might be changing your nail polish too often and drying the nails out with nail-polish remover.

Eliminate the obvious causes, then hydrate and seal in the moisture. This makes considerably more sense than paying the equivalent of up to $8 an ounce for tiny tubes or bottles of cuticle oil or nail conditioner. These products are simply not necessary.

Nail hardeners too have major flaws. The theory behind them is to artificially harden porous nails with formulas based on alcohol and formaldehyde, two preservatives that are perversely dehydrating. Nail hardeners actually do temporarily harden nails, but using them is, I think, absolutely the wrong approach to the problems of splitting or cracking. It's better to seek out and eliminate the causes of dryness. And if your nails are already damaged, cover them with nail polish, which is probably just as strengthening as any nail-hardening product. Again, I don't feel I can in good conscience recommend any specific hardening products, because I don't think you should buy them.

Nail Fortifiers

Nail fortifiers—a. k. a. "base coats" and "top coats"—are another hard coat over or under regular polish. They do indeed strengthen nails, but one wonders why they're marketed in a manner that undermines their credibility. To read the labels or listen to the cosmetic-counter girls who sell them, you'd think they were working chemical wonders on the fingernail itself. Not so. They fortify nails only because they provide an extra coating in addition to your regular polish. Two coats of polish will "fortify" your nails *just as well.*

Interestingly, a comparison of the ingredients in base coats and top coats reveals that they are the same product. It is true that using either (or both) along with regular nail polish will yield a deeper, more resonant shine. I wish the manufacturers would just say so, and leave it at that. Instead, we have expensive products like Clinique's ALLERGY TESTED BASE COAT and ALLERGY TESTED TOP GLAZE to contend with. For openers, the implication that Clinique alone tests for allergies is totally erroneous. Their tests are no more rigorous than the ones conducted on dimestore top coats. Next, we have the spectacle of attractive young women in white coats selling the product as if it were something that enhanced the health. Well, "Clinique" is not a clinic. Yet the dramatic aura that surrounds the Clinique counter manages to convince no small number of shoppers that that company's base coat and top glaze are worth nearly four dollars per half-ounce.

Save your money. You'll get equal results for a third of the price with either of these top two recommendations: L'OREAL MIRACLE ACCENTS MIRACLE BASE; or Revlon's WONDER NAIL NAIL FORTIFIER (despite the name). For slightly more, you can use either of a pair of equally good top coats from Revlon called EXTRA LIFE TOP COAT and SUPERSEALER. For a little more money (but still not too much) you can get equal satisfaction from Elizabeth Arden's VERY SPECIAL BASE COAT, Professional Cosmetics' ULTRAFINE NAIL-STRENGTH BASE COAT, Helena Rubinstein's STRONG & GLOSSY, Fabergé's LIQUID NAIL DRY, and ALMAY PROTECTIVE BASE COAT. If you find other reasonably priced base- or top-coat products where you shop, buy them with the knowledge that they offer no less than any of the luxury products by Chanel, Estée Lauder, Orlane, etc.

Cuticle Removers

Here's another item I don't like. Cuticles are there to protect the critical joining of the nail and the nail fold. Some people don't like the way they look, and for them the cosmetics industry has come up with these products.

O. K., chances are overwhelmingly in favor of your not having any adverse reaction to cuticle removers. They all work simply and similarly; you spread them on with a brush applicator, wait, then push the cuticle back with an orangewood stick. Are these removers a source of allergic reactions? Very rarely. Is it bad to remove the cuticle? I don't think it's a good idea, but lots of people do it and seem no worse for wear. Do cuticle removers prevent hangnails? Neither cuticles nor cuticle removers have anything to do with hangnails, which are irritatingly curved growths of the fingernail into the adjoining tissue. What is the name of a recommended inexpensive cuticle remover? MANI MAGIC CUTICLE REMOVER by the Leeming Pacquin division of Pfizer, Inc; it costs about 79¢ for three-quarters of an ounce.

What about those irritating little things that occasionally come out from under the edge of the nail (we'll call them "soft hangnails" for lack of a better term)? Whatever you do, *don't* pull them, or they'll hurt like crazy. The best approach is to clip them off as close as possible with a fingernail clipper, then tuck the end back under the nail as best you can. This is sometimes easier if you first soften them with Vaseline or another moisturizer before clipping and tucking.

FINGERNAIL PRODUCTS

Nail-Tip Whiteners

These are small white pencils used to color the under portion of the nail tips. The idea is to make manicured nails look cleaner and more attractive. I'm happy to report that nail-tip whiteners are cheap (less than 50¢), so you can experiment with their admittedly subtle effect without feeling profligate. They are also completely safe, which can't be said of everything. Whether or not you'll actually notice the effect is a moot point, but if small details like this are your thing, I recommend Revlon's NAIL TIP WHITENER and Flowery Manicure Products' FLOWERY PROFESSIONAL NAIL WHITE PENCIL. The pencils, incidentally, can be kept sharp with an eye-pencil sharpener.

CHAPTER 9

Hair Care and Coloring Products

Most people care intensely about the appearance of their hair, but they know next to nothing about it or about the products that purport to affect its growth and appearance. This lack of information has led to all manner of pseudoscientific misconceptions. People put the wildest things on their hair—weird shampoos, oils, and packs, things that effect no positive change and cost lots of money, to boot. To help alleviate this situation, I'm going to postpone product evaluations for a moment and first describe what hair really is and where it comes from.

Each human hair is a lifeless protein structure produced by an organ called a hair follicle. The average scalp has about 100,000 follicles, each of which is nestled into its own web of nutrient-carrying blood capillaries and buried well beneath the surface of the skin. Each follicle receives *all* its nutrition from the blood contained within its embracing capillaries. This is a point that should be kept in mind. Nothing that is applied to the surface of the scalp will affect the follicles below or the amount or quality of the hair they grow.

Hair grows according to a fairly regular three-part growth-and-shed cycle. Fortunately, our follicles are not synchronized, or we'd all go periodically bald. Instead, a varying number of follicles will at any given time be in the shed phase while others are in a rest phase and still others are actively growing hair. (Some mammals, incidentally, *do* have synchronized follicles. French poodles, for example, have an eighteen-year hair growth cycle, at the end of which *all* the hairs fall out. Most poodles don't live to that age, but those that do become completely bald, then start to regrow a new coat as their follicles reenter the growth phase.)

The three phases of the growth-and-shed cycle are called "anagen," "catagen," and "telogen." During the first of these, the anagen, or growth, phase, the most deeply buried part of the follicle embarks on a period of rapid metabolization. It becomes the scene of busy mitosis and cellular activity, and the deep end of the follicle begins to swell into a bulb. Like a little factory, it produces "keratin," the same protein substance that makes up fingernails. Like nails, the hair has no life of its own either; it's simply a byproduct of the metabolic activity taking place in the follicle. As long as this activity continues, the keratin keeps being produced and simultaneously formed into a hair shaft. And as more and more keratin is added to the shaft from the bottom, the shaft itself is gradually pushed up the narrow upper neck of the follicle, and eventually out of the follicle's surface opening. Throughout the anagen phase, the hair shaft continues to be pushed up from below and continues to get longer and longer.

Then suddenly, at a point that varies for each individual, the anagen growth phase ceases and the "catagen," or resting phase, begins. What stops anagen? Usually it's just a matter of the sort of follicles you've inherited. Some follicles have long and vigorous anagen phases; others don't. The anagen phase may be artificially terminated by strange diets that deny the body of basic nutrition (liquid protein has been shown to have this side effect); hormonal imbalances stemming from medication or from a physical or emotional trauma may also do it. Usually, however, the anagen phase just ends when your genes so dictate.

Catagen is called the resting phase because the follicle doesn't do anything. The rapid metabolism ceases, the bulblike enlargement of the follicle's deep end begins to shrink, and the hair shaft just rests in the follicle without any new keratin being added to its inner end.

The "telogen" phase commences when the hair shaft falls out of the follicle. The shaft isn't connected to anything, and it's not living, remember. As the follicle shrinks during the catagen phase, the hair becomes progressively looser; when it falls out, telogen has officially arrived at the follicle.

There are two kinds of hair loss: that due to follicles in the telogen phase and that which is permanent. You can expect to shed between 100 and 200 hairs daily from telogen follicles. That's normal and temporary, and the hairs will grow back when their follicles reenter the growth phase. It's also normal to temporarily lose hair after any sort of major physical trauma (like an auto accident), after pregnancy, during times of high emotional stress, or when starting or stopping a course of birth control pills. All these things can upset either the nutrient or the hormonal content of the bloodstream and prematurely kick an abnormal number of follicles into the telogen phase.

Permanent hair loss is another matter. It stems from follicles that have, in effect, gone to sleep. Follicles never die—even on a head as bald as a billiard ball. They still have the capacity to be reactivated, too, although no safe method has been found for it. Baldness is thought to depend on the amount of the male sex hormone androgen (or hormones similar in structure to androgen) in the bloodstream. As the body matures, more and more androgens and androgenic hormones usually accumulate. Depending on your follicles' inherited sensitivity to androgen levels in the blood, they will gradually start succumbing to the hormone and become inactive. One by one, the follicles reach the telogen phase, then simply never reenter anagen. How fast this happens, or whether or not this happens at all, is thought to be strictly a matter of the inherited level of resistance to androgen. The whole process is called "male pattern baldness," although it might just as well be called female pattern baldness. It afflicts both

HAIR CARE AND COLORING PRODUCTS

sexes, with the same thinning on the crown together with recession of the hairline at the temples. The effect, however, is mitigated among women, because female sex hormones (specifically, estrogen) tend to offset the effects of androgenlike hormones (like progesterone) in the female body.

There's absolutely nothing you can do to stop genetically caused male pattern baldness. Be stoical, or get a hairpiece. Whatever you do, don't waste money on products or treatments that promise renewed growth. Things applied to the scalp do nothing. Scalp massages have a similarly negligible effect. Neither approach affects either the capillaries surrounding the follicles or the blood they contain. The best thing you can do to insure healthy hair growth is simply to stay healthy and eat a balanced diet. The thinking behind "vitamins" for the hair is that bodies denied of certain vitamins will grow either poor-looking hair or no hair at all. The manufacturers imply that vitamin-deficiency conditions like this are prevalent. Actually, it's extremely rare for a normal person to lack enough vitamins for the condition to affect hair growth.

So much for the process of growing hair. What about the hairs themselves? What do they look like, how are they constructed, and how are they affected by hair preparations? Again and again the public is subjected to advertising that paints a wholly erroneous picture of hair. We are led to believe that a hair is a delicate living thing to be nurtured and cultivated. Actually, hair is dead and durable, and is not damaged without considerable effort.

Each hair has three layers—the "cuticle," the "cortex," and the "medulla." The outermost, the cuticle, is like a covering of overlapping shingles. If your "imbrications," meaning the spaces between the overlapping pieces of cuticle, are open, then the hairs won't lie neatly together or slide easily against one another when combed. Substances with an acid pH tend to close down your imbrications and thereby reduce friction and promote manageability. This is the logic behind acid conditioners and creme rinses, which we'll be discussing in detail. Substances with an alkaline pH tend to open the imbrications and fluff up the hair. This is why alkaline shampoos are attacked so mercilessly by advertisers. The fact of the matter, however, is that the opening of the imbrications caused by alkaline shampoos is so minimal and temporary that use of them in no way constitutes a threat to the condition of your hair.

The cuticle is your hair's first line of defense. It protects the layers below, and the hair's appearance is directly related to its proper maintenance. As the hair grows older—i. e. longer—the cuticle can become frayed and damaged and the imbrications permanently opened. This is what causes dull and unmanageable hair. If the cuticle is rubbed away altogether by overuse of harsh chemicals in hair products like dyes and permanents, the lower structures can begin to unravel. Result: split ends.

Just below the cuticle is the "cortex." Also made of keratin, the cortex is usually what's split in cases of split ends. There is pigment in the cortex, whereas there is none in the cuticle. There are also air bubbles, which determine the quality

HAIR CARE AND COLORING PRODUCTS

of your hair color by affecting the manner in which it reflects light.

At the very center of each hair shaft is the "medulla." Here's where most of the pigment is found. For hair dyes and permanents to work they must employ strong chemicals to penetrate the cuticle and cortex and get all the way down to the medulla. This process, especially when repeated regularly, is very damaging to the hair's outer layer.

When you come right down to it, it's amazing that so intricate a structure as a hair shaft, with so many structurally different parts, could be produced inside one little follicle. Furthermore, each of these parts is made from the same keratin, simply rearranged.

Now that you know the basic structure of hair, let me tell you just what can affect it and what can't. Since a hair shaft is dead, there is nothing you can apply to it to "nourish" it, or "moisturize" it, or perform on it any other organic-sounding function. The key to improving the appearance of the hair is simply to safeguard the condition of the cuticles. There are plenty of straightforward products on the market that do this very well. There is absolutely nothing baffling about choosing them, either—as long as you're well informed. The suggestion that only specially prepared products are safe enough for your hair is an erroneous hoax foisted on the public by the manufacturers of certain products. Everyone knows how frightened people are of hurting their hair. Manufacturers who try to make you feel like a dummy by smugly suggesting that good hair care is difficult and expensive are simply employing emotional blackmail.

Good hair care boils down to little more than a working knowledge of a few simple principles. Eating properly and staying in good health provide your follicles with everything they need to grow healthy hair. Avoiding traumas and shocks, insofar as possible, prevents temporary hair loss. Protecting the hair cuticles from destructive overuse of dye and permanent chemicals, blow driers, curling irons, sharp-toothed combs, and excessive brushing, helps keep hair shiny and manageable. Coating the hair with protein conditioners makes it look thicker and glues together ragged split ends. Using shampoo or soap to wash the hair every day opens the imbrications only slightly—enough to make the hair look fluffy, but not enough to hurt it. Adding oil (olive, mineral, or anything) to your shampoo will make dry hair easier to manage.

Throughout this chapter, I'm going to enlarge on these principles to give you a good working knowledge of the mechanics of hair care. I've organized my discussion around products in the following categories:

    Shampoos
    Conditioners
    Thickeners
    Hair Dressings
    Setting Lotions
    End Papers

SHAMPOOS

Hair Sprays
Anti-Gray Products
Bleaches
Dyes
Home Permanents
Facial Hair Bleaches

Shampoos

People too often forget that the purpose of shampoo is to clean hair. Shampoos aren't meant to provide protection from the environment, to repair damage to the individual hair shafts, or to make up for the deficiencies of overactive—or underactive—oil glands on the scalp, no matter what the shampoo manufacturers say.

Actually it's understandable that consumer expectations run so high on the subject. Shampoo labels promise the moon—and shampoo makers throw practically everything but that into their formulas. I'm speaking as a physician when I tell you that things like honey, wheat germ, peach juice, deionized water, skim milk, sage extract, and all the other vaguely healthful-sounding additives tossed in by creative shampoo formulators are pure window dressing. These kinds of additives have nothing to do with cleaning hair.

What cleans hair is soap. Plain old alkaline soap—or equally alkaline (if cheaper) synthetic detergent—is the skeleton in every shampoo formula's closet. And yes, every shampoo is also basically alkaline, despite misleading claims about "pH balance."

The manufacturers make such claims because alkaline substances like shampoo open the imbrications of the hair-shaft cuticle. But to suggest that this effect is minimized or eliminated by pH-"balanced" formulas is consumer deception of the slipperiest sort. The way these formulas are "balanced" is by simply adding enough acid to get a favorable reading on a piece of litmus paper. However, when one tests the pH of the *lather* formed by one of the "balanced" shampoos, it inevitably registers as alkaline. And the less alkaline it is, the less efficiently it cleans.

The silliest thing about all this is that there is nothing wrong with the alkalinity levels found in the average shampoo. O.K., alkalinity certainly does open the imbrications, *but* it does so only temporarily, and to a very limited degree. And in so doing it causes no damage to the hair shaft. What's more important, though, is that an alkaline substance like soap or synthetic detergent is the only thing that can effectively cut through the oily dirt on a head of hair.

Besides the useless fruit and vegetable additives mentioned above, there are many other adjunct shampoo ingredients that do a little good—but not much. My main objection to them is that they tend to obscure the shampoo's major function—to clean the hair. For example, the only difference among the many

HAIR CARE AND COLORING PRODUCTS

formulas for "oily," "normal," and "dry" (also referred to as "tinted" or "damaged") hair is just the amount of oil (like lanolin or mineral oil) added to the "dry" formula and omitted from the "normal" and "oily" varieties. Dry hair is a result of inadequate sebaceous oil on the scalp. Adding oil to the shampoo seems like a good idea, except that when you rinse out the lather, most of the added oil is going to go down the drain with the suds. The same can be said of the protein coating and conditioning agents found in many formulas. They provide a bit of coating and conditioning, sometimes that's all that's needed. But as soon as you rinse your hair, most of those added conditioners will be lost.

The key to coping with most problem dry or oily hair lies not in the shampoo you buy but in the way you use it. If your hair is too oily and looks matted or greasy, then shampoo more often and/or use more shampoo. There's no reason not to shampoo every day; shampoo's alkaline properties are simply not strong enough to hurt the cuticles of your hair. Lathering more than once won't hurt you, either, although it's really not necessary for cleaning most heads. If your hair is too dry and flyaway, then you should either shampoo less often, use less shampoo, and/or treat your flyaway hair with a conditioner (described in the next section). Just remember that shampoos are for cleaning, not for conditioning.

If your hair is limp, thin, and/or lacking body, you should also tackle the problem not with a shampoo but with a conditioner. This kind of hair still gets dirty and oily and still needs to be cleaned with shampoo. But, again, don't expect the shampoo to compensate for the hair's basic shortcomings. That's why conditioners were developed.

In fairness, I must note that nearly every shampoo on the market—misleading promotional claims notwithstanding—is harmless, easy to rinse, and won't cause tears. These products are formulated with great sophistication. In fact, the nearly universal high quality of most over-the-counter shampoos is doubtless the motivating force behind their often frantic efforts to distinguish themselves by making meaningless claims of pH balance and special formulas.

Because shampoos all have virtually the same soap and detergent bases, I advise you to buy either the least-expensive or best-smelling brand. Shampoos are truly unisex cosmetics, too; there's simply no way to differentiate the hair-cleaning needs of men from those of women. The hair is the same; it's exposed to the same environment; the same shampoos work with equal effectiveness for either sex.

I'm sure there are lots of readers who remain convinced that their special hypoallergenic, pH-balanced, nonalkaline shampoo is (as their hairdresser told them) the *only* thing to use on their sensitive, delicate hair. To this I say, fine, if you have a shampoo you really like, then keep using it. I'm sure that whatever it is, it's just as good as my own favorite, PRELL (in liquid or concentrate form). Prell, however, has the advantages of being inexpensive and widely available. I

SHAMPOOS

also highly recommend FLEX BALSAM AND PROTEIN SHAMPOO (by Revlon), L'OREAL SHAMPOO (normal, dry, tinted, or "preference" formulas), ALBERTO VO 5 GENTLE AS RAIN WATER SHAMPOO, and JOHNSON'S BABY SHAMPOO, as well as all the discount drughouse-brand shampoos (that bill themselves as anything from "herbal" to "organic" to "pH balanced"), and, for that matter, plain soap. The virtue of these products is their low price. They all clean hair every bit as safely and effectively as the most esoteric shampoos from Clinique or Pantene. Don't be a price snob; it's absolutely O. K. to buy cheap shampoo.

As to the advisability of shampoos that contain special conditioning or coating agents, I think they help—but only a little. If your hair needs conditioning, you should use a conditioner and not depend on a shampoo. But if you use both a conditioning shampoo and a separate conditioner it won't hurt. The following list contains a number of dependable shampoo brands together with notes on their special additives and claims. These are all pleasant enough products and I don't hesitate to recommend them—on the basis of their cleaning ability, not because of their additives.

As for nice-smelling shampoos, I can only give you my personal preferences.

ADDITIVES IN SHAMPOOS

Shampoo brand	Special Additive(s)	What the Additives do
Alberto Balsam Shampoo (by Alberto Culver Co.)	balsam	this dark brown, viscous liquid is an oily conditioner derived from the tree of the same name
Clairol Herbal Essence (by Clairol, Inc.)	hydrolized animal protein	a coating agent to promote body and manageability
Clairol Short & Sassy (by Clairol, Inc.)	gelatin citric acid	the gelatin is a coating agent; the acid helps close the imbrications of the cuticle
Everynight Balsam & Protein Shampoo (by Helene Curtis)	balsam protein	balsam helps with dry-hair problems and protein coats the shafts for added body and shine
Fabergé Organics Pure Wheat Germ Oil & Honey Shampoo (by Fabergé, Inc.)	allantoin calcium pantothenate (plus a lot of useless wheat germ and honey)	these first two additives are chemical coating agents
Ionax Shampoo for Oily Hair & Scalp (by Owen Labs)	sodium laureth sulfate	a chemical detergent similar to those found in regular shampoos

Continued

HAIR CARE AND COLORING PRODUCTS

Cont.

Shampoo brand	Special Additive(s)	What the Additives do
Pantene Shampoo for Fine or Thin Hair (by Pantene Co.)	hydrolized animal protein	a coating agent
Pernox Shampoo for Oily Hair (by Westwood Pharmaceuticals)	sodium laureth sulfate lactic acid hydrolized animal protein	the first two are detergent degreasers; the protein is a coating agent added for manageability
Protein 21 pH Balanced Shampoo (by Mennen Co.)	hydrolized animal protein citric acid	the protein is a coating agent; the citric acid helps close down opened imbrications
R-gen Protein Hair Repair Shampoo (by Owen Labs)	hydrolized animal protein	a coating agent
Redken Genuine Amino Pon Shampoo (by Redken Labs)	hydrolized animal protein (plus a number of other proteins) formaldehyde	all the proteins are coating agents; the formaldehyde is a preservative (that often causes allergic reactions)
Revlon Milk Plus Six Shampoo & Conditioner (by Revlon, Inc.)	milk protein	a coating agent
Wella Balsam Conditioning Shampoo (by Wella Corp.)	balsam	an oily conditioner meant to help dry and/or unmanageable hair

I'll unblushingly recommend certain shampoos on the basis of smell because I know they will also clean perfectly well. Sometimes the creative cosmetic urge seems to have gotten lost between the kitchen and the laboratory, as in the case of FABERGÉ'S PEACH A LA MODE MILK PROTEIN SHAMPOO WITH NUCLEIC ACID which sounds as if it might explode. Other good-smelling products include:

    CLAIROL SUNSHINE HARVEST SHAMPOO (by Clairol, Inc.)

    "GEE YOUR HAIR SMELLS TERRIFIC" SHAMPOO (by Andrew Jergen Co.)

    EVERYNIGHT HERB SHAMPOO (by Helene Curtis)

Similarly, the good-smelling products of Vidal Sassoon, Almay, Yves St. Laurent, Aramis, Brut, etc., are all perfectly good cleaners. They're worth their price if you appreciate their scent.

SHAMPOOS

I don't think much of shampoos whose manufacturers carry on about their supposed ability to pamper your hair. Hair doesn't need to be pampered, at least not with shampoo. Somewhere along the way everyone seems to forget that shampoo is for cleaning and not for the repair of damaged hair. The ads also often seem to imply that shampooing with other formulas is a typical source of hair damage. And this is not true. So for these reasons, I don't think much of CLINIQUE HERB SHAMPOO (with its pretentious hair-improvement claims and high price tag), DHS DERMATOLOGICAL HAIR AND SCALP SHAMPOO (which is ordinary shampoo masquerading as some kind of special dermatological concoction), PURPOSE SHAMPOO (marketed as if its ordinary protein additives make it something particularly suited for men who use blow driers). Most of these products are expensive, too. I can say only that they do clean hair at least as well as Prell.

Finally, we have dandruff shampoos—a category in which medicine and cosmetics have finally made a good marriage. Dandruff is a type of psoriasis, a skin condition wherein the rate of skin-cell turnover is unnaturally accelerated. The result of this overly fast turnover is the accumulation of little white flecks of dead skin.

Dandruff looks like hell, so it's fortunate that there are several different and equally effective approaches to keeping it in check. The first of these employs the application of tars to the affected skin area. Tars are obtained from the destructive distillation of pine, coal, or any organic material. They are dark and viscous, antiseptic and deodorizing, and also carcinogenic under certain conditions. When applied to the scalp in any antidandruff-formula shampoo, they are not thought to pose any cancer threat. Instead, they slow down the rate of cell multiplication, thereby relieving the cause of the dandruff.

Two other chemicals have the same effect. These are zinc pyrithione and selenium. Like tars, these chemicals affect the metabolism of the skin cells in a way that seems to slow down the rate at which they shed from the surface.

Another antidandruff approach employs peeling agents to effectively strip away the top layers of dead cells before they can collect in showers of unsightly flecks. The most popular peeling agents used in dandruff shampoo are sulfur and salicylic acid, substances that are also widely used in antiacne therapy.

Since the human body has a knack for rapidly getting used to medicines—and thereby reducing their effectiveness—the key to using dandruff shampoos is to switch around. Use one for a while, then change to another. Don't stick with the same product, because the longer you use it the less effective it will become. The lists below divide the most popular dandruff shampoos into active-ingredient categories. If your dandruff is mild, an occasional shampoo with any one of the recommendations will probably take care of it. If your problem is persistent, buy small bottles of different brands and use a different one each morning.

HAIR CARE AND COLORING PRODUCTS

Recommended Tar-based Antidandruff Shampoos

*IONIL T NONIONIC/CATIONIC THERAPEUTIC DANDRUFF SHAMPOO (by Owen Labs)

*IOCON SHAMPOO TAR GEL CONCENTRATE FOR DANDRUFF CONTROL (by Owen Labs)

POLYTAR SHAMPOO (by Stiefel Labs)

SEBUTONE THERAPEUTIC TAR SHAMPOO (by Westwood Pharmaceuticals)

TEGRIN MEDICATED SHAMPOO (by Reedco, Inc.)

Recommended Antidandruff Shampoos Based on Zinc Pyrithione or Selenium

ZINCON DANDRUFF SHAMPOO (by Lederle Labs; with zinc pyrithione)

HEAD & SHOULDERS SHAMPOO (by Procter and Gamble; with zinc pyrithione)

SELSUN BLUE (by Abbott Labs; with selenium)

Recommended Antidandruff Shampoos with Sulfur and/or Salicylic Acid

SEBULEX MEDICATED SHAMPOO (by Westwood Pharmaceuticals; with both)

VANSEB DANDRUFF SHAMPOO WITH PROTEIN (by Herbert Labs; with both)

IONIL NONIONIC/CATIONIC THERAPEUTIC DANDRUFF SHAMPOO (by Owen Labs; with salicylic acid)

Conditioners

There's a very good chance that you don't need a conditioner at all. Only if your hair is dry and difficult to comb, or drab and lusterless, or filled with unsightly split ends, or thin and in need of added fullness, will you definitely benefit from using one.

The effect of any conditioner is limited and temporary. I think many consumers are misled by the implication (contained in many advertisements) that a conditioner will permanently set to right whatever's ailing your hair. Of course, the

---

* Works well but smells bad; follow it with an additional lathering with a more aromatic general-purpose shampoo.

truth of the matter is that a lifeless hair shaft can't possibly be "healed." All the conditioner in the world won't restore damaged hair to its original condition. What it does—and does well—is cover up the damage.

Conditioners operate within a limited framework. They can coat hair shafts with protein, thereby temporarily glueing split ends back together and giving each hair shaft a bit of extra thickness. They can close the cuticle imbrications with acid ingredients, and closed imbrications make the hair look shinier. Smooth cuticles also increase manageability by cutting down on the electrostatic charge caused by friction. The oils in conditioners can also supplement an insufficient level of oil produced by the sebaceous glands on the scalp. The additional oil can make the hair both easier to comb and shinier.

If your hair is long, there's a better than even chance that you really *do* need a conditioner. This is because long hair is old hair, and old hair is more prone to what could be called mechanical damage to the cuticle. Long hair has been exposed for a longer period time to shampoo detergents, weather, combing, and brushing, to any bleach or dye chemicals you may have tried, and especially to cuticle-wrecking blow driers, curling irons, and other heating appliances. All these things slowly wear away at the cuticle. Even if your cuticles are strong and thick, some degree of normal wear is inevitable. And the longer you wear your hair, the more obvious this natural wear will become.

Incidentally, there is no cure for split ends. They must be cut off. The protein ingredients in many conditioners, however, can go a long way in masking a split-end problem and keeping it from becoming noticeable until you have the hair cut.

The same protein that glues split ends together can also give your hair the appearance of added thickness. Of course, nothing's going to make the hair actually start growing in more thickly, but protein conditioners make what you have look bulkier and thicker. Besides thickening each shaft, a protein coating makes the individual shafts stand apart more, slide better against one another, and shine.

Many people turn to conditioners because their hair is drab. But sometimes hair drabness is a symptom of a systemic disorder. Iron deficiency anemia (the sort that tonics like Geritol are aimed at) is a common cause of drab hair. So is thyroid deficiency. You may also be taking certain serious drugs that can affect the hair—for instance, certain of those used in cancer therapy. In cases like these any conditioner is clearly unequal to the task.

However, if your hair is drab and difficult to comb purely from a lack of natural lubricating scalp oil, a conditioner may be just the thing. With its acid-induced shine, protein coating, and lubricating oils, a simple after-shampoo conditioner may readily solve your problem.

I'm a firm believer in using conditioners separately from shampoos. As noted earlier, there are many shampoos that contain conditioning ingredients, and there is even a newer species of product called the "shampoo-conditioner." These do

HAIR CARE AND COLORING PRODUCTS

work to a certain degree. But I can't believe that very much of any conditioner applied to and rinsed from the hair along with shampoo soaps and detergents can adhere to the hair shafts.

You should always apply conditioner to freshly shampooed hair. But how long do you leave it on? The assumption in some minds is that the longer you leave it on, the more of it will stick to the hair shafts. This seems logical, except that if you compare the formulas of "instant" hair conditioners to those meant to be left on the head for thirty minutes or so, you'll find that there is hardly any difference between them. I think that about two minutes is adequate time for most any conditioner to do what it's going to do. Remember, conditioners are not working chemical miracles on your hair shafts, nor are they stimulating subtle metabolic changes or growth processes. They're just coating the hair. Personally, I think that after five minutes, any conditioner will have done its best.

How about the difference between "conditioner" and "creme rinse"? If a distinction can be made at all, it would be based on the amount of protein in the formula. Creme rinses should really be called acid rinses, because they are often simply an acid substance meant to be combed through the hair to close the imbrications and promote shine and manageability. Conditioners usually contain protein ("hydrolized animal protein" is the overwhelming favorite; it's just a highly processed and refined protein) that is meant to be massaged into the hair. Creme rinses typically contain protein ingredients as well as acids, and conditioners usually contain some acid ingredients. So it's hard to make a sharp distinction between the two.

Many people condition their hair with home recipes that often work nearly as well as commercially prepared products. For example, lemon juice is a good, simple creme rinse whose natural acidity closes up the imbrications on the hair shaft. This makes combing easier, and gives the hair shine thanks to the smoothed cuticles. Egg whites are natural protein substances (as opposed to fatty egg yolks) and combing them through the hair, then rinsing the excess with water will coat the shafts and help add body. (Incidentally, beer, a carbohydrate with a very iffy smell, does nothing for the hair. Generations of women have used it, but that doesn't mean it coats hair shafts or increases shine and manageability. Remember, doctors used leeches for centuries before they were abandoned as useless.) I'd compare the effectiveness of home conditioning with acids, proteins, or even oils to that of shampoo-conditioners. They do help, but not as much as a separately applied, commercially prepared conditioner/creme rinse formula. The commercial products are more thoroughly processed; for that reason the proteins they contain will adhere better to the hair shafts, the acids will be better distributed through the hair by the other ingredients and the oils will be sufficient to lubricate without leaving the hair unpleasantly greasy.

When you buy a conditioner, you're really buying a very simple and nonmysterious combination of acid, protein, and oil, all bound together in a pleasant-smelling base. The following list contains recommended body- and shine-inducing conditioning products that are reasonably priced, widely available, and designed to be applied to freshly shampooed hair (towel drying is optional), and rinsed out in one to five minutes:

AGREE CREME RINSE & CONDITIONER (by Johnson Wax Co.)

ALBERTO VO 5 WHIPPED CREME RINSE & CONDITIONER (by Alberto Culver Co.; in an aerosol can)

AQUAMARINE CONDITIONING CREME RINSE ("Regular" and "Extra Body" formulas; by Revlon, Inc.)

BEAUTIFUL HAIR BRECK CREME RINSE (by John H. Breck, Inc.)

BRECK BEAUTIFUL HAIR CLEAN RINSE (by John H. Breck, Inc.)

CLAIROL HERBAL ESSENCE CREME RINSE (by Clairol, Inc.)

CLAIROL INSTANT CONDITION TREATMENT (by Clairol, Inc.)

EARTH BORN pH BALANCED CREME RINSE & CONDITIONER (by Gillette Co.)

FLEX BALSAM & PROTEIN INSTANT HAIR CONDITIONER (in "Super Concentrated Regular," "Penetrating Conditioner for Damaged Hair," and "Creme Rinse" formulas; by Revlon, Inc.)

LONG & SILKY CONDITIONING LOTION FOR LONG HAIR (by Clairol, Inc.)

PROTEIN 21 CONDITIONER (by Mennen Co.)

SHORT & SASSY CONDITIONING LOTION (by Clairol, Inc.)

TAME CREME RINSE & CONDITIONER (also in "Lemon Fresh" and "Extra Body" formulas; by Gillette Co.)

WELLA GENTLE CARE INSTANT HAIR CONDITIONER ("Regular" and "Extra Body" formulas; by Wella Corp.)

If you don't have thick hair, then *don't* use any of the products on the list that follows. These add oils (usually mineral oil, petrolatum, lanolin, balsam, etc.) to normal or thick hair that is dull and difficult to manage.

CARYL RICHARDS: BALSAM PLUS PROTEIN INSTANT HAIR CONDITIONER (by Fabergé, Inc.)

DEP BALSAM MIST PROTEIN HAIR CONDITIONER (by DEP Corp.)

FABERGÉ ORGANICS: PURE WHEAT GERM OIL & HONEY CONDITIONER (by Fabergé, Inc.)

NESTLÉ BALSAM PLUS VITAMIN E INSTANT HAIR CONDITIONER (by Nestlé-Lemur Co.)

HAIR CARE AND COLORING PRODUCTS

SUAVE: BALSAM & PROTEIN INSTANT HAIR CONDITIONER (by Helene Curtis)

WELLA BALSAM INSTANT CONDITIONER (by Wella Corp.)

WELLA IN-DEPTH CONDITIONING TREATMENT FOR PROBLEM HAIR WITH PROVITAMIN B 5 AND PROTEIN (by Wella Corp.)

Some of the products on this last list are meant to be rinsed out and others aren't. Some also contain important-sounding ingredients—like Vitamin E, honey, and "provitamin B 5"—that have absolutely nothing to do with the condition of your hair shafts. However, all of them contain lubricating oils, are reasonably priced, and have an attractive scent, which is why I recommend them.

Several other conditioners bear mention. Even though I don't think there's much point to leaving any conditioner on the hair for longer than five minutes, some people like the ritual of a conditioning beauty pack. CLAIROL CONDITION BEAUTY PACK TREATMENT is nice stuff, and the directions have you keep it on for thirty minutes. If you like it, fine; it's got plenty of protein. WELLA KOLESTRAL tells you to keep it on (preferably under a plastic cap) for five to fifteen minutes, and it too has protein aplenty.

One of the most damaging things you can do to your hair cuticles is to submit them to daily treatments with hot blow driers, curling irons, and, to a lesser degree (because they're not as hot as blowers and irons), hot rollers. The heat from these appliances causes cumulative scorching damage to the cuticles. Use them enough, and you'll leave your imbrications permanently fried open (result: a dull, unmanageable thatch), or you'll wear the cuticle off entirely (result: split ends). Despite the long-term damage they wreak, hairstyling gadgets that reshape hair by means of heat remain popular. If you use one, you really must also use a protein-coating conditioner before each session. And, instead of rinse-out conditioners, I recommend that you use those that are meant not to be rinsed. The last three products on the list below are designed specifically for use with blow driers. But any one of the six will afford the cuticle at least some measure of protection.

HAIR SO NEW CREME RINSE (by Clairol, Inc.)

KINDNESS INSTANT PROTEIN HAIR CONDITIONER (by Clairol, Inc.)

BRECK BASIC: CONDITIONER WITH PROTEIN (by John H. Breck, Inc.)

PRE HEAT PROTECTIVE CONDITIONER (by Andrew Jergen Co.)

CLAIROL POWER PAL CONDITIONING STYLING MIST FOR BLOW DRYING (by Clairol, Inc.)

HEAT SOLUTION DE PANTENE (by Pantene Co.)

How about hair that's been submitted to the rigors of an antidandruff shampoo? Dandruff shampoos are very drying, so a lubricating conditioner is certainly in order. There are even a couple of products designed specifically for this purpose. Two good ones are IONIL RINSE CONDITIONER (by Owen Labs) and SELENE INSTANT HAIR CONDITIONER (by Abbott Labs). But, in point of fact, any product with oily balsam, mineral oil, or lanolin is just as good as Ionil or Selene.

Finally, a word about conditioners for black people. The structure of blacks' hair differs from that of whites primarily in the cortex layer of the hair shaft. This contains air bubbles that affect the way the hair reflects light. In black people these air spaces are arranged so as to produce a natural matte finish. Aside from that—plus a typical flatness of the shaft that accounts for curliness regardless of race—the structure of the hair is essentially identical to that of whites.

Because of the general structural similarity of their hair, black people can and usually do use the same hair products as whites. If more shine is desired to offset the natural matte finish, either a dressing or one of the oily-type conditioners already mentioned can be used. The Johnson Products Company of Chicago has cornered the market for black people's conditioners. The following are sold under the tradename AFRO-SHEEN: an oily HAIR SPRAY, which is really just a dressing intended for use on dry hair; a CONDITIONER AND HAIRDRESS, which is a similar concoction of lanolin, mineral oil, and petrolatum and is also applied as a dressing; a MEDICATED CONDITIONER AND HAIRDRESS that contains sulfur to combat dandruff as well as the same oil ingredients above; and something called COMB EASY HAIR CONDITIONER LOTION, which contains acetic acid (a. k. a. vinegar) to close up the imbrications and induce shine. As a group, these products are fairly oily. They also straddle the line between hair dressings (more about which later) and conditioners. Unless you like the look of very shiny hair, I'd stick with the more nondenominational recommendations above.

Thickeners

Thickeners are supercoating conditioners whose application gives the illusion of added fullness to a head of hair. You apply them to clean, damp hair, comb or brush it into place, allow it to dry completely, then comb or brush the dried hair a last time to fluff it up.

If you feel your typical hydrolyzed animal protein or gelatine-based conditioner isn't adding enough body, a thickener is definitely worth a try. They are aimed subliminally at men fearful of balding. But, of course, they work equally well for women, since everyone has the same hair. They work best (that is, give the apperance of greatest thickness) for those who have at least a moderate amount of hair.

How do they do it? With vinyls and special waxes! Interesting to note, one

HAIR CARE AND COLORING PRODUCTS

of the waxes contained in THICKET (by Madric Ltd.), an expensive but quite effective thickener, is "carnauba" wax. You may perhaps recognize it as an ingredient in certain automobile polishes. Still and all, Thicket easily washes out of the hair with tomorrow's shampoo.

Less expensive and applied in the same way is THICK 'N HAIR (by Fantasia Industries Corp.). It's just as safe, just as easy to wash out, and often just as effective, at about a fifth the cost of Thicket). My advice: if you're interested, buy a small tube or bottle of each and experiment.

Hair Dressings

These products are styling aids that keep the hair in place. Like thickeners, you apply them sparingly to freshly shampooed, towel-dried hair, which is then combed or brushed into place, allowed to dry completely, then often combed one last time to give a fluffier, more full-bodied look. Then, presto, you're ready to meet the world.

Sometimes the label tells you that washing the hair before application is optional. I say that hair with any natural accumulation of oil (and probably yesterday's dressing if you haven't washed it since then) is not going to look grand. It'll look greasy. Dry-look products as well as traditional oily preparations build up quickly. My advice is to apply them only to clean hair that's still slightly damp. That way you won't lose fullness because of matting from too much natural oil plus that in the dressing. The dampness will help distribute the dressing evenly.

The two major families of hair dressings—the dries and the oilies—have formulas based either on variations of alcohol or of oil. Alcohol dries and hardens. Oil (I can't bring myself to call it grease) just sits there and glistens. I don't know of anything in any hair dressing that could hurt anybody. They're all safe, and they all work. But the look they give you is a little too neat and controlled for some tastes.

Personally, I much prefer the dry products, because I think dry hair looks more attractively natural. It looks fuller, too. Speaking of fullness, don't expect any hair dressing to give it to you. Dry products work best for people with lots of thick normal or oily hair. They cause a certain amount of matting (not as much as the oil-based dressings), but that doesn't matter if you have a lot of hair. What's in a typical dry formula? Things like "sulisobenzone," "triisopropanolamine," "stearalkonium chloride," and similarly unpronounceable alcoholic drying substances. The following list contains a half-dozen recommended dry-type dressings.

    DEP DRY STYLING CONTROL (by DEP Corp.)
    VITALIS DRY TEXTURE FOR MEN'S HAIR (by Bristol Myers Co.)
    VITALIS CLEAR GEL GREASELESS HAIR GROOM (by Bristol Myers Co.)

HAIR DRESSINGS

> VITALIS WITH V 7 (by Bristol Myers Co.)
>
> THE DRY LOOK LIQUID HAIR CONTROL (by Gillette Co.)

No matter what the product is called, each and every one is as suited for women as it is for men. The same can be said of the oil-based products in the list below. Oily dressings have been so out of favor lately that I was amazed to discover so many of them still on the market. Again, they're meant to be applied to clean, damp towel-dried hair, then combed. They differ from the dry products because there's no alcohol to evaporate. Oil-based dressings—they contain things like mineral oil, beeswax, propylene glycol, petrolatum, and lanolin—work best on thick, dry hair that has plenty of body, but that needs a bit of oil-induced shine and manageability. The following is a list of recommended oily dressings arranged in ascending order of oiliness:

> SCORE MICRO-EMULSION HAIR GROOM (by Bristol Myers Co.)
>
> GILLETTE HEADS UP HAIR GROOM (by Gillette Co.)
>
> GROOM & CLEAN GREASELESS HAIR CONTROL (by Chesebrough-Pond's Co.)
>
> BRYLCREEM AND BLUE BRYLCREEM FOR GREY HAIR (by Beecham Products)
>
> PROTEIN 29 HAIR GROOM (by Mennen Co.)
>
> WILDROOT CREME OIL (by Colgate Palmolive)
>
> VASELINE HAIR TONIC AND SCALP CONDITIONER (by Chesebrough-Pond's Co.)
>
> ALBERTO VO 5 CONDITIONING HAIRDRESSING (by Alberto Culver Co.)

A few footnotes: Score is good stuff, but the term "micro-emulsion" signifies nothing about the product's effect on human hair. I like Groom & Clean too, but you'd be foolish to expect it to perform any kind of real cleaning function. (The label says "rinses grease, dirt and dandruff out of your hair . . . in the shower.") Blue Brylcreem is blue because of the addition of an intensely blue liquid called "azulene." One school of thought holds that gray hair looks better when tinted blue. Protein 29 has cuticle-coating hydrolyzed animal protein and cuticle-smoothing citric acid in its formula and so is almost a conditioner. Alberto VO 5 is the oiliest product on the list; it does wonders to transform a thick, dry thatch into a lustrous mane.

A last word on dressings: if you're a dandruff sufferer, you might want to augment your antidandruff shampoo with an antidandruff dressing. The following pair of recommendations are both good oily-type products, use of which won't

HAIR CARE AND COLORING PRODUCTS

hurt your hair even if you don't have dandruff. The first is PROTEIN 29 CREME HAIR GROOM (by Mennen Co.), which contains sodium pyrithione; the second is green-formula BRYLCREEM (by Beecham Products) with zinc pyrithione. These two chemicals retard the skin-cell turnover rate and thereby help to control dandruff flaking.

Setting Lotions

Setting lotions are normally used in conjunction with rollers or pin curls, and their purpose is to help hold a set. (Of course, the simplest setting lotion is plain water.) Put damp hair in a roller, let it dry in position, and you'll have formed a curl. The additional application of setting lotion to the damp hair will make the curl stronger, longer lasting, and more resistant to curl-relaxing humidity.

Setting lotions won't damage the hair, because they don't affect either the cuticle or its imbrications. All they do is coat the hair, usually with variants of alcohol and vinyl plastics. In fact, they're very similar to hairsprays, except that they're cheaper and a little more time consuming to apply.

Most setting lotions now come in pump-spray dispensers. You shampoo and rinse, spray the lotion liberally onto wet or towel-dried hair, depending on the directions, comb through, then put in your rollers or pin curls. After the hair dries, the curls are gently combed or brushed out. The following list contains my favorite pump-type setting lotions, each of which works very well and is reasonably priced.

REVLON PROFESSIONAL SETTING LOTION (by Revlon, Inc.)

L'OREAL NATURALLY FREE SETTING LOTION (by Cosmair, Inc.)

L'OREAL SATINE SETTING LOTION (by Cosmair, Inc.)

GET SET SETTING LOTION (by Alberto Culver Co.)

OGILVIE CONDITIONING SETTING LOTION (by Tussy Cosmetics)

Setting lotions can be used along with conditioners—as a separate step, of course. Some lotions even contain conditioning ingredients like hydrolyzed animal protein and citric acid. Frankly, I think these chemicals are superfluous. They won't hurt you, but there's not enough of them in any setting formula to really help hair that needs conditioning. Use these products for their holding abilities; don't expect them to do much else.

Two other good setting lotions in the pump-spray form are marketed primarily as hair sprays. These are CLAIROL FINAL NET (by Clairol, Inc.) and FLEX NON-AEROSOL HAIR NET (by Revlon, Inc.). You can spray either of these onto dry hair that's already been styled, but you can also spray them onto wet hair as a setting lotion. They work very well.

Even though I think the pumps are easiest to use, two other nonpump products deserve mention. These are BRECK SET SETTING LOTION (by John H. Breck, Inc.) and WELLA FLEX SETTING LOTION (by Wella Corp.). Both are very strong-holding products that come in squeeze bottles and are highly recommended.

Setting "gels" are simply setting lotions in a nonliquid form. The method of application—combing through clean, damp hair—is the same for all brands, and so is the effect. I recommend the following pair of gels for their effective holding power and sensible price.

> DIPPITY-DO SETTING GEL (formulas by Gillette Co.; regular and extra-hold)
>
> BALSAM DEP SUPER HAIR STYLING GEL (by DEP Corp.)

Question: What's the difference between "regular" and "super-hold" setting lotions? Answer: The "super" formula contains more alcohol or plastic, as the case may be.

Question: Is there any holding ingredient worth a premium price tag? Answer: In my opinion, no. Setting lotion ingredients are drawn from a fairly short list of alcohols and plasticizers. It's certainly not worth paying a premium for added conditioning ingredients. The only reason I can see for the high price on products like SET DE PANTENE (by Pantene Co.) is to promote an image of exclusivity.

Question: Can setting lotions be used to straighten the hair? Answer: Yes, indeed they can (only temporarily, of course). One product in particular, L'OREAL HOLD STRAIGHT (by Cosmair, Inc.), is advertised as a straightener, even though it can just as easily be used to set curls. The way to remove, or at least help minimize, unwanted curls with setting lotion is to thoroughly permeate the shampooed hair with the product, wind the hair onto very large rollers, let dry, and comb out.

End Papers

They come in packets containing up to a thousand individual tissue-type papers. And they make curls smoother while preventing wispy and crushed ends. End papers are designed to be used with rollers on hair that is clean, damp, and treated with setting lotion if desired. The paper is wrapped around the base of each group of hairs to be rolled, then slid down the shafts until the ends are covered. The covered end is then put onto the roller, rolled up, and allowed to dry.

LADY LORA END PAPERS (by Lady Lora Co.) are inexpensive and work perfectly. They are representative of the simplest end paper, namely, the type that is untreated. You may also buy end papers that have been treated with setting solution. The dampness in your hair unlocks the solution, which then imparts added hold

HAIR CARE AND COLORING PRODUCTS

to your curls. I think treated end papers are a good idea, and I especially recommend WET AND SET TREATED CURL PAPERS (by H. Goodman & Son, Inc.).

Although it's not an end paper, I'll recommend another product here, since it also helps makes set hair smoother: SCOTCHBRAND HAIRSET TAPE (by 3M Co.) is convenient and versatile and very easy to remove. You can use hairset tape for all sorts of other things—like setting wigs, holding bangs and sidecurls in place until set, taping your own hair under a wig, keeping long hair from becoming tangled in bed overnight, etc.

Hair Sprays

These are more products that help hold a set. They can be used with setting lotions and/or treated end papers, or in place of them. You'll have to decide just how many of these holding aids your hairstyle requires.

Hair sprays fall generally into two categories: those based on alcohol (for a soft hold); and those based on plastics and vinyl resins (for a strong hold). Women's hair sprays come in both varieties, whereas hair sprays "for men" are almost all soft-hold alcoholic formulas. Once again, there is absolutely no reason for a woman not to use a man's hair-spray product if she likes it. And if you are a man with a complicated hairstyle, there is also absolutely no reason not to use a woman's strong-hold formula.

As of this writing, fluorocarbon propellants have been almost, but not quite, eliminated from hair sprays as a group. The aerosol cans are now usually powered with things like carbon dioxide, which works so well you may wonder why anybody ever even bothered with those treacherous fluorocarbons. A spinoff of the fluorocarbon controversy has been the proliferation of pump sprays. These make much more sense, I think, because they give you many more applications per can than aerosols, regardless of the propellant.

Do strong-hold formulas make the hair look lacquered? Well, very often they do. But that's just the price you'll have to pay if you want a head full of intricate and carefully positioned swirls. The trend in hair fashion at the moment is away from this kind of look, but there are still plenty of hair sprays that'll help you achieve it if you want it. The following list contains recommended products based on vinyl resins, related plastics, and complicated esters and acetates. Since I like pumps, I'll recommend those first.

Strong-hold Sprays in a Pump

    FLEX NON-AEROSOL HAIR NET (by Revlon, Inc.)

    FINAL NET (by Clairol, Inc.)

    MISS BRECK: LASTING HOLD NON-AEROSOL HAIR SPRAY (by John H. Breck, Inc.)

HAIR SPRAYS

> WELLA-FLEX HAIR NET (by Wella Corp.)
>
> VIDAL SASSOON NON-AEROSOL HAIR MIST (by Vidal Sassoon, Inc.)

Neither the products above, nor any of those that follow, will hurt your hair. They all just coat it temporarily, then wash right out with the next shampoo. The products on the next list of recommendations also contain strong-hold resins, plasticizers, and the like, except they're marketed in aerosol cans instead of pump sprays.

Strong-hold Sprays in an Aerosol

> ALBERTO VO 5 MIRAL PLUS HAIRSPRAY FOR IMPROVED HOLDING (by Alberto Culver Co.)
>
> CARYL RICHARD'S JUST WONDERFUL HAIRSPRAY (by Fabergé, Inc.)
>
> PROTEIN 21 HAIRSPRAY (formulas by Mennen Co.; regular and extra hold)
>
> L'OREAL SUFFRAGE HAIR SPRAY (by Cosmair, Inc.)
>
> ALMAY HAIR MIST (by Almay, Inc.)
>
> HAIR SPRAY DE PANTENE (by Pantene Co.; reasonably priced, too!)

Now, what about the hair sprays without the plastics? Well, these are all based either on alcohol or some close chemical cousin. The most common ingredient is something called SD alcohol 40 ("SD" means "specially denatured" or undrinkable), which, incidentally, is also contained in most of the strong-hold formulas. Soft-hold spray formulas hold hair in a manner rather similar to dry-look hair dressings. In other words, as the alcohol evaporates, it hardens the curls into position. Frankly, I prefer the soft look obtained from these products. And since I also prefer pumps, I'll give you my soft-hold-in-a-pump recommendations first.

Soft-hold Sprays in a Pump

> ALBERTO VO 5 NON-AEROSOL HAIRSPRAY (by Alberto Culver Co.)
>
> THE DRY LOOK PUMP SPRAY (by Gillette Co.)
>
> GILLETTE MAXI HOLD SUPER HOLDING HAIR SPRAY (by Gillette Co.)
>
> VITALIS REGULAR HOLD (formula by Bristol Myers Co.; also in Super Hold)

HAIR CARE AND COLORING PRODUCTS

You'll note that most of these are products "for men." But they're excellent for women too, so keep them in mind if you want to try a soft-hold pump. As for the occasional claims of "super holding," just put them down to promotional hyperbole. If you really want super holding, stick with one of the vinyl- or plastic-based sprays above.

The next list contains good aerosol sprays of the soft-hold variety. Like the pump products, they're usually based on SD alcohol 40. And again, I haven't separated men's from women's products because there is no medical reason to do so.

Soft-hold Sprays in an Aerosol

>ADORN SELF-STYLING HAIR SPRAY (by Gillette Co.)
>
>ALBERTO VO 5 HAIRSPRAY (by Alberto Culver Co.)
>
>ALL PURPOSE AQUA NET PROFESSIONAL HAIR SPRAY (by the Rayette division of Fabergé, Inc.)
>
>CONSORT HAIR SPRAY FOR MEN (by Alberto Culver Co.)
>
>DEP FOR MEN DRY STYLING HAIR CONTROL (by DEP Corp.)
>
>BRYLCREEM SOFT HAIR (by Beecham Products)
>
>PROTEIN 29 HAIR GROOM (by Mennen Co.)
>
>PROTEIN 29 DRY CONTROL FORMULA (by Mennen Co.)
>
>SCORE NATURAL HAIR SPRAY (by Bristol Myers Co.)
>
>DRY LOOK (by Gillette Co.)
>
>VITALIS DRY 3 HAIR CONTROL (by Bristol Myers Co.)
>
>BRUT 33 HAIR CONTROL SPRAY (by Fabergé, Inc.)

Anti-Gray Products

The following preparations are based on safe, nontoxic metallic dyes, and they're a good alternative to regular hair dyes that contain high levels of controversial (and possibly carcinogenic) coal-tars. Anti-gray products are also easy to use and won't damage the hair shafts—and, as we'll see, you can't say that about regular hair dyes.

Anti-gray products are massaged into the hair like a hair dressing, then either rinsed out or not. The darkening effect is gradual, and, since application is easy to control, you're able to limit the areas you want to darken. This makes it easy to keep a bit of distinguished gray, at the temples, for example.

There are a few drawbacks, such as the range of colors, which is very limited. You can't go blond or auburn; all you can do is darken gray hairs so that they no longer contrast with your natural color. You must also sharply curtail your shampoo and grooming habits during the initial period of use. (Once a week, maximum, for shampoos, and no grooming or setting products at all until you achieve the desired darkening effect).

How long does it take to get rid of the gray? The exact answer depends on the color and texture of your hair, but several weeks is average. Once you hit the desired shade, you can return to your normal shampoo and grooming regimen and reapply your anti-gray formula only when new hair growth necessitates it.

YOUTH HAIR in liquid or cream form (by Majestic Drug Co.), RD in lotion, cream, or shampoo (by L T Laboratories), and GRECIAN FORMULA 16 (by Coombe, Inc.) in lotion or cream, are all dependable anti-gray preparations designed for use by both men and women. They really work, and they come with detailed instructions. For people whose hair looks terrible unless shampooed daily, let me especially recommend the RD shampoo. With whatever product you use you'll get permanent color that won't wash out. Exposure to sunlight, incidentally, enhances the darkening effect.

Bleaches

Just as safe as the metallic anti-gray dyes—and a good deal easier to use—is simple hydrogen-peroxide bleach. Hydrogen peroxide for the hair is just a stronger concentration of the drugstore disinfectant of the same name. When applied to the hair it opens cuticle imbrications (none too gently, either) and oxidizes the natural melanin coloring substance contained within each hair shaft. There's nothing carcinogenic about peroxide, and it's cheap and effective. For these reasons it's one of the best ways to change hair color.

Peroxide is also used in conjunction with the dye chemicals discussed below. It helps dye get past the protective cuticle so it can effectively bind itself to the inner structure of the hair shaft.

In both home- and salon-dye products, the peroxide is called the "developer." CLAIROXIDE LIQUID DEVELOPER (by Clairol, Inc.) is therefore labeled as if it were only suitable for use with Clairol's line of permanent dyes. Actually, it's an excellent and very inexpensive bleacher that can be used all by itself to lighten hair without the addition of coloring agents. The following list contains more recommended bleaches. These differ from Clairoxide inasmuch as they contain added conditioning ingredients to minimize and smooth cuticle damage. I don't think added conditioners help very much, but they make these products a little nicer to use—and more expensive.

ULTRA SILK HAIR LIGHTENER (by Revlon, Inc.)

SNOW SILK LIGHTENER (by Revlon, Inc.)

BORN BLOND LIGHTENER (by Clairol, Inc.)

HAIR CARE AND COLORING PRODUCTS

    SUMMER BLOND (by Clairol, Inc.)

    YOUNG BLOND (by L'Oreal—Cosmair, Inc.)

    LEMON GO LIGHTLY (by Clairol, Inc.)

I don't know how lemons got their reputation as a hair lightener (note the name of the last product above), because they have no effect on hair color. Since lemons are acidic, they actually close hair imbrications—which is not the effect you want when bleaching hair.

Sunlight, on the other hand, definitely does help lighten hair, the more so when it shines on hair still damp with peroxide solution. If you can't languish by a sunny pool while bleaching your hair, a sunlamp is a good alternative. Hold the lamp above you, keep it moving slowly, limit exposure time to no more than a minute or two with each peroxide treatment, and beware of exposed skin lest you get a sunlamp burn.

Dyes

A great controversy is currently raging as to whether or not hair dyes cause cancer. What are the facts? The evidence is incriminating but far from conclusive. Hair dyes certainly don't pose the same threat as cigarette smoking. But they may very well have more carcinogenic potential than saccharin, for example.

Way back in 1938, hair-dye industry lobbies were successful in exempting dye chemicals from regulation by the Food and Drug Administration. Since then, the exempted chemicals—and especially those that give darker shades of color—have been eliminated from all foodstuffs because of their known carcinogenicity. The assumption has always been that putting them on your scalp is not the same as eating them. Certainly this seems to have been the general public's perception, since sales of hair dyes continued to rise despite the bad publicity.

However, substances applied to the skin are now known to be absorbed into the system. That includes carcinogenic hair-dye chemicals. The industry points out that the cancer controversy stems from experiments on rats forced to absorb the equivalent of two dozen bottles of dye per day. On the surface, this would seem to discredit the whole idea of testing with rats. However, these tests (conducted by the National Cancer Institute) allow for the rat's lifespan of only a few years. The high dosages are an attempt to adjust for the human life of many more years, during which a person could expose himself to great quantities of dye chemicals. Some people argue that if you feed anything to a rat in such large dosages, it will be bound to cause cancer. However, the Cancer Institute tests included nine control substances administered in dosages equal to that of the suspect dyes. None of the controls caused cancers. Finally, industry defenders have noted that there is no statistical correlation between women who use hair dyes and women who have cancer. Unfortunately, cancers often take decades to develop. Hair dyes have been in wide use only about twenty years. It may be another twenty before any correlation between use and the incidence of cancer becomes apparent.

How, then, can you evaluate the chance you may be taking by using a hair dye? First of all, if there is *any* history of cancer in your family, I advise you to dispense immediately and entirely with dyes. Whether the evidence is inconclusive or not, it's simply not worth the risk if you might have inherited a predisposition to cancer. Next, you can avoid using dark dyes, which contain more potentially carcinogenic chemicals. Those that caused cancer in rats are listed on dye labels as 4-MMPD (s) or 2,4-DAA (s). If you use dye, it's almost impossible to entirely avoid these chemicals, but you can lessen your contact with them by using paler shades. A safer course would be to give up dyes completely and stick with peroxide or anti-gray formulas.

There are three basic types of hair-dye products that employ suspect dye chemicals: permanent dyes; semipermanent dyes; and temporary tints. Permanent dyes involve complicated multistep procedures, and you are well advised to have them applied professionally—at least the first time. The permanents are the dyes that employ a peroxide developer to penetrate the hair shafts to bind permanently to the inner structure of the hair. The color you get won't wash out, but, of course, you'll have to keep reapplying it to cover new growth. Constant reapplication of peroxide developer is the sort of thing that permanently opens imbrications, causes split ends, and inhibits manageability. It used to be that the dye, the developer, the plastic gloves, and the mixing bottles all had to be purchased separately for home hair coloring. But now you can buy complete kits with everything you'll need, as well as detailed instructions on how to use it all. I think CLAIROL'S NICE 'N EASY and L'OREAL'S PREFERENCE are the best of the prepackaged kits. As an alternative, you can buy your developer, etc., separately, and choose your specific color from the many lines of dyes on the market. MISS CLAIROL HAIR COLOR BATH CREME FORMULA and CLAIROL BALSAM COLOR, EXCELLENCE EXTRA RICH HAIR COLOR and PREFERENCE (by L'Oreal—Cosmair, Inc.), TRIED AND TRUE (by Max Factor), FANCI-TONE (by Roux), and BRECK HAIR COLOR (by John H. Breck, Inc.) are examples of comprehensive lines of hair dye to be used with peroxide developers.

Semipermanent hair dyes substitute chemicals like sulfur and ammonium thioglycolate for peroxide. They fade and wash out with a few shampoos, but application is somewhat easier than with permanent dyes, and the absence of peroxide means less damage to hair cuticles. On the other hand, semipermanent coloring is still a lot of work and mess for a less than lasting effect. And, although the hair-softening chemicals used to promote color binding are milder than peroxide, they are not *good* for your hair.

I don't think much of semipermanent dyes. They seem like more work than they're worth, which is why I can't wholeheartedly recommend semipermanent products like SILK AND SILVER COLOR LOTION (by L'Oreal—Cosmair, Inc.) or LOVING CARE COLOR FOAM, HAPPINESS, or LOVING CARE HAIR COLOR LOTION (all by Clairol, Inc.).

HAIR CARE AND COLORING PRODUCTS

Temporary color tints or rinses are my least favorite coloring products. They contain neither peroxide nor sulfur nor thioglycolate. But, even though they won't hurt cuticles, they must be reapplied so often that there's a constant threat of dulling buildup. They also wash right out in a single shampoo—or a cloudburst, if you're unlucky enough to be caught in one. And they rub off on collars and pillows. If you're going to dye your hair at all, you might as well use a permanent dye product. It may be more trouble at first, but continual reapplication of temporaries or semipermanents eventually becomes just as much trouble. And the same possible carcinogenic dye chemicals are present in all three forms.

FANCI-FULL RINSE (by Roux), NESTLÉ PROTEIN COLOR RINSE and NOREEN COLOR RINSE HAIR (by Nestlé) and PICTURE PERFECT COLOR RINSE (by Clairol, Inc.) are typical of the many temporary color rinses on the market. I don't recommend any of them.

Frankly, my advice is to avoid dyes. I know the cancer case isn't completely conclusive, but I for one am convinced. If you want to change the color of your hair, you're far wiser either to bleach it with peroxide and sunlight, treat it with an anti-gray formula, or use the ancient reddish tint called HENNA. This last product has been used by women for literally thousands of years. It is completely safe and organic (derived from the leaves of an African bush), coats the surface of the hair (thereby adding body and shine), doesn't involve peroxide (or any other harsh chemicals that soften the cuticle or open the imbrications too much), and is cheap. Henna is manufactured in this country by the Hopkins Company. It's applied either as a paste or a rinse, left on for varying amounts of time (depending on how much red you want), then shampooed out. The biggest drawback to henna is its color limitation. The possibilities range from auburn to reddish brown—only. There is also an occasional problem with buildup from repeated applications, but, on balance, that's a low price to pay for the convenience, safety, and efficacy of henna.

Home Permanents

How do these ingenious products work? First, let me say that they work the same in a beauty salon as they do at home. And as with hair coloring, there's a lot of technique and expertise involved in getting good results. That is why I strongly recommend that your first permanent be done by a professional.

The primary active ingredient in permanent-wave solutions is thioglycolate, the same chemical that enables Nair to dissolve hair elsewhere on the body. The difference between the waving solution and a bottle of Nair is merely one of concentration; when used on the head, a weaker solution of thioglycolate will soften the hair and help it accept its new position on a roller without undue damage. The application period is closely timed and promptly followed by a water rinse and a hydrogen peroxide neutralizer. After the softening action is terminated, the hair is allowed to dry in position. Salons often apply heat at this point to further reinforce the new curled position. Home permanents are often just left to dry after neutralizing, but using a blow drier on your rollers produces a curl-enhancing effect.

Do home permanents work well? The answer is yes, at least as long as you carefully follow the directions and know how to place your rollers. But, if you leave the waving solution on too long, you'll risk a rotten case of split ends or extensive breakage at the scalp line. If you don't leave the solution on long enough, the permanent might not take. There's also the question of proper application of the crucial neutralizer. If applied too late, or too sparingly, you'll risk the same damage caused by overapplication of waving solution. And, of course, if it goes on too soon, it'll terminate the permanenting before the hairs fully accept their new position.

Are there any particular dangers to home permanents? No, actually they're pretty safe. They don't contain suspected carcinogens, and even if you were to really damage your hair with overapplication, there is some comfort in knowing that the follicles would not be affected, and that the damage would eventually grow out. As for allergic reactions, there's always somebody who'll have one. If it happens to you, rinse the affected area with neutralizer and cool water at once, and apply soft cloths soaked in the soothing compress mixture described at the end of the Introduction.

Let me reiterate my advice that you go to a professional for your first permanent. Home permanent packages have detailed instructions, and lists of what you'll need, but they are simply no substitute for watching a professional—especially when it comes to proper roller placement. Once you get the knack of it, there's no reason not to give yourself future permanents. I give an equal recommendation to TONI (by Gillette Co.) in "gentle home," "super home," and "advance look" varieties, and to L'OREAL EXTRA BODY PERM (by L'Oreal—Cosmair, Inc.)

Facial Hair Bleaches

These products offer an alternative to often expensive and uncomfortable methods of hair removal such as electrolysis, Depilatron, or waxing. They bleach the color from unwanted hair on the face (and arms, too) thereby rendering the hair unnoticeable. The products listed below are each safe and simple to apply. About the only preparation needed is a brief washing with soap and cool water (to close the pores). After that the bleaching product is mixed with its accelerator, or activator, applied with a spatula, left on for five to fifteen minutes (depending on instructions), then scraped away with the spatula and rinsed. The following products get my equal recommendation:

JOLEN CREME BLEACH (by Jolen, Inc.)

AIME LIPBLEACH (by Aime Mfg. Co.)

BLONDIT (by MEM Co.)

NUDIT CREAM BLEACH FOR THE FACE (by Helena Rubinstein)

CHAPTER 10

Acne Preparations

It may surprise you to learn that the most common cause for a visit to the dermatologist by a fully grown adult is none other than an acne breakout. Acne, the scourge of adolescence, is often perceived as a problem that one "grows out of." Not so. It's a problem whose cause lies in excessive secretion of oil on the surface of the skin. And this is a problem that is just as likely to plague an adult as a teenybopper.

What leads to an acne breakout is hormonally induced enlargement of the sebaceous oil glands located just below the surface of the skin. These glands sometimes open into sweat ducts (pores), sometimes into hair follicles, and sometimes surface by themselves in the middle of an otherwise hairless, ductless patch of skin.

The heaviest concentration of oil glands is on the face, but they are also located in lesser concentrations everywhere on the body. The oil they produce is the body's natural moisturizer. It provides a barrier against the evaporation of water and helps the skin stay supple. People who don't have sufficiently active oil glands are the ones who must use moisturizers.

Oil glands that secrete *too much* sebaceous oil, however, can clog the surface openings of the skin. Excessive oil secretion is either caused by oil glands that have been hormonally stimulated to enlarge (as, for example, in adolescence), or by oil glands that have been hormonally stimulated to overproduce oil (as in many cases of emotional stress), or by both. The biggest oil-gland stimulant is the male sex hormone androgen. But the body can be easily "fooled" into the same hyper oil production by substances that are merely *like* androgen. For example, the adrenal glands of both sexes produce a wide range of androgenlike steroid hormones, many of which are released into the bloodstream at times of physical danger or emotional stress. These hormones can very often lead to acne flareups. And although female bodies don't produce androgen, they do produce an androgenlike sex hormone called progesterone. Contained in certain birth control pills, this hormone may also trigger breakouts.

Many foods are highly androgenic, and eating them really increases your chances of acne eruptions. Wheat gluten of the sort used in gluten bread and certain meat substitutes, as well as the health-food favorite wheat germ are prime examples. Other substances have a molecular structure that is so similar to androgens that they, too, can cause excessive oiliness. A common example is iodine. Some studies have linked acne breakouts with fast food, not because of the deep fats and oils used in the cooking, but because of the iodine used to sterilize the cookers. It seems that enough iodine gets into the food to actually cause acne eruptions among consumers of Big Macs, Whoppers, Whalers, etc. Spartan health-food faddists are no safer, since kelp, sea salt, saltwater fish, seaweed, and cabbage all contain significant amounts of iodine. As for those who tread the middle ground between junk food and health food, be advised that shellfish, artichokes, peanuts, and most multivitamins have just as many potentially acnegenic iodides as the foods listed above.

Many people suspect soft drinks, candy, cheese, fatty foods, and especially chocolate of causing acne. Only one of these has actually been shown to have an acne connection; that's soft drinks—and *only* soft drinks that contain brominated vegetable oil or other bromides (which are very similar to iodides). Sugar, long a suspect, has no connection to the body's production of sebaceous oil. The same goes for chocolate, cheese, and fatty foods; they have no impact on your oil glands at all, and no relation to acne.

Acne-causing substances in the diet just simulate acnegenic hormones in your own body. In adolescence, the body produces androgens and androgenic hormones for the first time. The result is excessive oil production and attendant breakouts. Among adults, stressful life situations often have the same effect. Stress wreaks havoc on the hormonal balance of the bloodstream and in medical circles is considered your skin's worst enemy. Too much adrenalin (from anything from a lost job to an uncertain love interest) can overwork your oil glands like a heavy burst of teenage androgen.

Besides diet, hormones, and stress, certain medicines cause acne by stimulating oil production. The cortisone in many poison-ivy treatments is one such drug; others are INH, used to combat tuberculosis; dilantin, used in therapy against seizures; the phenobarbitol in certain asthma and diet drugs; and the iodides in many cough medicines.

How Do Pimples Form?

Whatever its origin, a surfeit of skin oil does two things: (1) it provides a good, rich diet for the bacteria that normally live on the skin's surface; and (2) it can clog up pores, follicles, and/or oil-gland openings. Under normal circumstances, skin bacteria are quite harmless. They go about their metabolic processes without bothering a thing, at least as long as you keep your skin clean and its openings unclogged. But if you become too oily and can't keep your pores open, you may have a problem. You see, skin oil that has been acted upon by bacteria is chemically changed in a manner that makes it rather irritating. And if, due to excessive oil production, the irritating oil is trapped inside a follicle or pore

ACNE PREPARATIONS

or oil-gland opening, it will irritate the surrounding tissue. If the oil plug isn't removed the irritation will grow and eventually attract white blood cells ready for combat. Result: an inflamed and swollen pimple filled with white blood cells (a. k. a. pus).

The main thrust of OTC (over-the-counter) acne therapy is to dry up excessive oil, promote a bit of surface peeling to dislodge incipient oil plugs, and to provide mild antibacterial action. The good news is that most OTC acne medicines do this very well. The ones that are especially good are those that contain benzoyl peroxide, a drying, antibacterial degreasing agent that until very recently was available by prescription only.

Let there be no mistake about how acne medicines work. They do not *cure* pimples, they merely clean up the affected area and reduce the concentration of bacteria. This helps lessen the chance of more pimples developing, but in no way will it speed the healing of existing pimples. Let me also add that it's hard to be sure exactly what makes pimples go away. Many people attribute dramatic improvements in their acne to products that might well have had nothing whatsoever to do with it.

Acne Medicines

The four products named here are my favorite OTC acne preparations. Benzoyl peroxide alone is the active ingredient in each; no additional active ingredients are present to complicate matters.

> OXY-5 ACNE LOTION (by the Norcliff-Thayer division of Revlon, Inc.)
>
> CLEARASIL ANTIBACTERIAL ACNE LOTION (by Vick Chemical Co.)
>
> ACNE CREAM (by the Cuticura division of Purex)
>
> LOROXIDE ACNE LOTION (by Dermik Labs)

A few benzoyl peroxide products are still sold by prescription only. In some cases this is because they have a higher concentration of the active ingredient (often 10% instead of the customary 5%); sometimes the prescriptions contain the same 5% concentration, and why they remain prescriptions is absolutely a mystery. The following 5% products are practically identical to the nonprescription items above.

> 5-BENZAGEL and 10-BENZAGEL (by Dermik Labs; the latter has a 10% benzoyl peroxide content)
>
> DESQUAM-X 5 GEL and DESQUAM-X 10 GEL (by Westwood Pharmaceuticals; again, the latter has twice the amount of benzoyl peroxide)

ACNE MEDICINES

PANOXYL-5 GEL and PANOXYL-10 GEL (by Stiefel Labs; same concentrations as above)

SULFOXYL LOTION REGULAR and SULFOXYL LOTION STRONG (by Stiefel Labs; again, in 5% and 10% strengths)

PERSA-GEL 5% and PERSA-GEL 10% (by Texas Pharmaceuticals)

BENOXYL-5 LOTION and BENOXYL-10 LOTION (by Stiefel Labs)

There is no difference in the effectiveness of lotions, cream, or gel in either prescription or nonprescription products. The different forms are made solely to suit the whims of acne-product consumers.

Acne products in general—and especially those with benzoyl peroxide—are extremely drying. They're made primarily for extra-oily teenagers, so, when adults use them, there's a chance that some areas of the skin may become too dry. If you are not overly oily but still suffer from adult acne, be sparing with these products. Apply them only to the affected areas. And don't be afraid to use them in conjunction with a moisturizer if you need to.

Because adult skin is normally less oily than that of teenagers, I recommend a trio of very good, mild acne lotions that treat existing breakouts, provide a measure of protection against future acne flareups, and do so without turning your mature skin to parchment. The first is NEUTROGENA ACNE DRYING GEL pH6, a simple concoction of isopropyl alcohol and witch hazel. It's pure, it's natural, it strips away surface oiliness, and, if you'll overlook the pH6 nonsense (which has no bearing on its performance), I think you'll find it effective. The other two products, praised by patients of mine who say they feel good to the touch and are not excessively drying, are KOMED ACNE LOTION and MILD KOMED ACNE LOTION. Both contain salicylic acid and resorcinol, two oil-stripping antibacterial agents, as well as drying isopropyl alcohol and germicidal sodium thiosulfate. The "mild" formula contains lower concentrations of everything but the alcohol.

Resorcinol, which is a widely used antibacterial and astringent agent contained in Komed as well as in many other acne products, presents a danger for black people. Resorcinol can *very often* stain black skin darker. For white people, these acne medicines work well to adequately degrease the skin and deplete its surface bacteria count without undesirable side effects. But black people should beware the following acne medicines as well as any others that contain resorcinol:

CLEARASIL ACNE PIMPLES CREAM MEDICATION (by Vick Chemical Co.)

PHISOAC CREAM (by Winthrop Labs)

REZAMID ACNE LOTION (by Dermik Labs)

BARE-FACE (by Pennwalt Pharmacraft)

ACNE PREPARATIONS

Benzoyl peroxide has recently supplanted sulfur as the OTC treatment of choice for drying up acne-prone areas of the skin. Still, many products either contain sulfur or are based almost wholly upon it. Recently, Dr. Albert Kligman of the University of Pennsylvania conducted tests that cast doubt on the efficacy of sulfur. What's worse, his test results suggest that sulfur, the treatment of choice for acne for all these years, might actually be a *cause* of acne, by paradoxically promoting oiliness. Dr. Kligman's studies are not absolutely conclusive, but significant doubt has now been cast on sulfur's role in acne therapy. Even though the jury is still out on the matter of sulfur, you should keep this controversy in mind. The following preparations contain significant amounts of sulfur:

>   CLEARASIL ACNE PIMPLES CREAM MEDICATION (by Vick Chemical Co.; also contains resorcinol)
>
>   FOSTRIL DRYING LOTION FOR ACNE (by Westwood Pharmaceuticals)
>
>   PHISOAC CREAM (by Winthrop Labs; also contains resorcinol)
>
>   FOSTEX CM (by Westwood Pharmaceuticals)
>
>   REZAMID ACNE LOTION (by Dermik Labs; also contains resorcinol)
>
>   KLARON ACNE LOTION (by Dermik Labs; also contains resorcinol)
>
>   SULFACET-R LOTION (by Dermik Labs)
>
>   SULFOXYL LOTION (by Stiefel Labs; regular and strong formulas)

What about acne soaps? First, very many of them are manufactured with traditional sulfur therapy in mind. Like the preparations mentioned above, acne soaps are intended to degrease the skin, to promote a bit of peeling, and to be antibacterial. And Kligman's studies notwithstanding, there are still many proponents of sulfur therapy. The following acne soaps contain sulfur:

>   SASTID SOAP (by Stiefel Labs)
>
>   SULFUR SOAP (by Stiefel Labs)
>
>   SALICYLIC ACID AND SULFUR SOAP (by Stiefel Labs)
>
>   ACNE-AID DETERGENT SOAP (by Stiefel Labs)
>
>   ACNAVEEN (by Cooper Labs)

MULTI-SCRUB (by Bristol Myers; in liquid or cream form)

BUF (by Riker Labs)

FOSTEX (by Westwood Pharmaceuticals)

Sulfur seems to work for some people, but take note: if one of these products doesn't work for you, then *none of them will*. And, considering the Kligman experiments, I'd personally steer away from sulfur.

Besides, there are other products to wash with if you like this approach to acne therapy. I think LISTEREX LIQUID (by Warner-Lambert, with salicyclic acid) is excellent; so is IONAX FOAM (by Owen Labs, with benzalkonium chloride); IONAX SCRUB (by Owen Labs, with benzalkonium chloride plus little scrubbing granules similar to beauty grains); LISTEREX CLEANSING GEL (by Warner-Lambert, with thymol); PROPA pH (by Bio Products, with boric acid, thymol, and benzoic acid); CLEARASIL MEDICATED CLEANSER (by Vick Chemical Co., with salicylic acid); and NEUTROGENA ACNE CLEANSING SOAP (by Neutrogena Corp., with thriethanolamine lauryl sulfate). Like sulfur, these active ingredients are all antibacterial degreasers that are slightly drying.

Oil control is the name of the game in acne, and there are various other things you can do to control yours. You can wash your acne-prone areas several times daily with soap and water. Soap won't hurt your face, and it's excellent for removing excess oil and grease. You can also use any alcohol-based astringent for spot application to extra-oily areas. Cotton swabs or Q-tips dipped in alcohol, astringent, or witch hazel, and regularly applied to these areas are often just as effective as more costly acne preparations. Sun exposure is also good for acne, because it makes the skin peel a little, which has the effect of stripping away incipient oil plugs.

If you have troublesome acne, I advise you to medicate yourself in moderation. The older you are, the less your skin can tolerate the extreme drying effect of medicines with benzoyl peroxide, salicylic acid, or, for that matter, plain alcohol without becoming uncomfortably dry. Use a little at a time and limit application to just the affected areas. Since it makes no difference, from a medical standpoint, whether you use soaps, creams, scrubs, liquids, or gels, use whatever form suits you best. And remember that whatever you use, it'll probably make you feel a bit too dry the first day. This is nothing to be concerned about, since your skin will usually adjust itself to the product in a day or so.

If you consult a dermatologist about your acne, he may very well take a different approach and put you on a course of antibiotics. The favorite of these is tetracycline, a prescription pill that attacks the skin bacteria responsible for metabolizing harmless sebaceous oil into irritating acnegenic oil. Many people now hesitate to take pills, however, and for them there are a variety of topically applied antibiot-

ACNE PREPARATIONS

ics. Although not F.D.A.-approved yet, it looks as if topically applied antibiotics are the wave of the future in acne therapy. Doctors are presently writing prescriptions for them in some cities, particularly for topical erythromycin. They may well be available everywhere soon.

Should You Squeeze Pimples?

Yes! Emphatically! Squeezing pimples and blackheads will *not* cause more of them to appear. It *will* hasten the healing process by untrapping irritating skin oil and cornered bacteria.

Just be sure you're careful in cleaning out the pimple. Otherwise you *will* make it worse. Unsuccessful squeezing can force the irritating oil farther into the surrounding tissue, causing more tissue irritation and bringing more white blood cells to the site.

The best way to squeeze a pimple is with a little drugstore item called a comedo extractor ("comedo" is the medical term for pimple). The extractor looks something like a dentist's tool with a point at one end and a tiny spoon with a small hole in it at the other. The idea is to nick off the head of the pimple with one end, then press the spoon against the pimple to squeeze out the contents. If you didn't already know, this is exactly what professional cosmetologists do at sleek big-city skin salons. Comedo extractors are available in quality pharmacies; check Chapter 15 for brand-name recommendations.

CHAPTER 11

Products for the Feet

The overwhelming majority of foot problems fall into three categories: foot perspiration and attendant odor; fungus infections (usually called "athlete's foot"); and calluses.

Perspiration and Odor

Let's look first at foot odor, an uncomplicated if embarrassing problem for millions. What causes it? The same thing that causes odor anywhere else on your body: when you perspire, the bacteria on your skin take the perspiration, metabolize it (that is, "eat" it), and leave behind odoriferous byproducts.

Foot perspiration occurs at an unnatural rate on almost everybody, because feet weren't meant to be enclosed all day in hot shoes. But, interestingly, even though shoes are a setup for excessive sweating, most foot-odor problems stem from the type of bacteria that happen to live on your skin. Whether or not yours are of a type that produces strong odor is purely a matter of luck. And whether or not your odor problem is acute, it will usually respond well to the same approach used on underarms—to dry up and/or retard perspiration with anti-perspirants, and/or kill off odor-producing bacteria with antibacterial deodorants.

The simplest approach is usually the best, I think. That's why I recommend JOHNSON & JOHNSON DEODORANT FOOT POWDER in a spray can as my number-one choice for feet with problem perspiration odor. The simple formula is based on modified cornstarch, which, like all powders, soaks up wetness, helps keep the problem area dry, and so deprives bacteria of perspiration to metabolize. This product also contains alcohol and menthol, both of which impart a cooling, refreshing sensation. Alcohol is also mildly antibacterial. What's more, the product is cheap, another compelling reason for putting it at the top of the list.

In Chapter 4, I described how deodorants and anti-perspirants work. To recapitulate briefly: deodorants contain substances that kill odor-producing bacteria; anti-perspirants contain aluminum salts, which reverse the electrical charge of

PRODUCTS FOR THE FEET

the sweat ducts and impede the flow of perspiration. The result of the latter process is to deprive surface bacteria of perspiration to metabolize. "Anti-perspirant deodorants" simply combine both approaches in one not-necessarily-superior formula.

Deodorant and anti-perspirant foot sprays work in exactly the same way. If you need more odor protection than that found in a simple cornstarch powder like Johnson & Johnson's, I'd recommend an antibacterial deodorant foot spray. (By the way, you can just as well spray your feet with your underarm deodorant. It will work as well there as it does on your underarms, though it probably won't contain the cooling menthol found in so many foot products.) I prefer an antibacterial deodorant over an anti-perspirant because it's simpler and more direct.

Another favorite foot deodorant is QUINSANA DEODORANT FOOT POWDER. This pleasant powder is based on perspiration-absorbing talc, to which triclosan (the same antibacterial found in many deodorant soaps), silica (for smoothness), and an attractive scent have been added. It's a nice, straightforward product without the sort of unnecessarily complicated formula that characterizes some of its competitors.

Quinsana gets first place, but a quartet of other foot deodorants jointly share second:

Product name	Antibacterial ingredients
SCHOLL FOOT DEODORANT SPRAY	methylbenzethonium chloride zinc phenolsulfonate
DR. SCHOLL'S FOOT POWDER	boric acid
SCHOLL'S DEODORANT REFRESHER SPRAY	methylbenzethonium chloride zinc phenolsulfonate
JOHNSON'S FOOT SOAP	borax iodine

Note that Dr. Scholl's Foot Deodorant Spray is almost identical to the Refresher Spray. Why the latter costs almost twice as much as the deodorant is a mystery to me. Both products contain chemical bacteria killers that are considerably stronger than the boric acid in Dr. Scholl's Foot Powder or the iodine and borax in Johnson's Foot Soap. I like the foot soap because it feels so good to use—even though washing each foot separately isn't so convenient.

JOHNSON'S ODOR EATERS (from the same company that makes the foot soap) represent another concept in foot-odor fighters. These are deodorant insoles you slip into your shoes; you get three pairs to a package. The active agent in the insole is something they call "miracle activated charcoal," which sounds as if it belongs in a cigarette filter. Many studies show that charcoal traps odors, but I don't think this product can do that much for your feet. The approach seems after the fact in my mind; better to kill odor-producing bacteria with deodorants or to inhibit excessive perspiration with anti-perspirants than to leave the cause of the odor problem unattended while you cram another insole into your shoe.

Now for the foot anti-perspirants: in Chapter 4 I was hard pressed to find any distinctions among the underarm anti-perspirants, because they all work on the same principle and contain the same active ingredient. Well, we've got the same situation here; the foot anti-perspirants all contain aluminum salts and all are equally effective. Medically speaking, there are hardly any grounds to differentiate them.

Since I like the cooling feel of menthol in a foot spray, I'd give my top recommendation to the following two sprays: DRI-FOOT DEODORANT SPRAY AND ANTIPERSPIRANT and GILLETTE FOOT GUARD, FOOT DEODORANT AND DRY SPRAY POWDER. Both these products also contain a little something to kill off bacteria—plain alcohol in the case of Dri-Foot, and triclosan in Gillette Foot Guard. But their primary thrust is to reverse the polarity of sweat ducts in the skin of the feet by means of aluminum salts.

Other effective aluminum-based products include QUINSANA FOOT DEODORANT SPRAY POWDER ANTIPERSPIRANT; SCHOLL DRY ANTIPERSPIRANT FOOT SPRAY; and DR. SCHOLL'S BROMIDROSIS FOOT POWDER. Dr. Scholl also puts together something called DR. SCHOLL'S CHLOROPHYLL FOOT DEODORANT POWDER, which seems to contain everything but the kitchen sink. Besides aluminum chlorhydrate, the formula includes talc, bentonite (a chalky, drying substance favored in some acne preparations), zinc stearate, and sodium copper chlorophyll (an antibacterial). This is a complicated concoction, and, unless you're a real connoisseur of foot sprays, I'd advise you to stick with something simpler.

If foot perspiration becomes unmanageable, you can develop a condition called "dyshydrosis." This is symptomized by extremely uncomfortable little blisters, which usually appear on the sides of the feet. People who suffer from dyshydrosis—also known as the "sweaty sock syndrome"—have feet that sweat so profusely the perspiration literally can't all make it out of the skin. Instead, it collects in the blisters, which break, become irritated, and often contribute to embarrassing odor problems. The best treatment for dyshydrosis is a simple talc or cornstarch powder to soak up the wetness, together with zinc oxide paste (a drugstore item) to soothe the irritation. If you do develop dyshydrosis blisters, you are well advised to wear shoes that allow your feet to breathe more freely.

Fungus Infections (a. k. a. "Athlete's Foot")

Fungi love warm, dark, moist places, which is why they love to attack sweaty feet. And when they do, they cause the itching discomfort known as "athlete's foot." Perhaps you've wondered just how contagious athlete's foot really is. Unfortunately, there is no simple answer to this question. Some people seem to have a predisposition to fungus infections—just as certain individuals always seem to catch colds. At the same time, there are others who can stamp barefooted through public showers all day long and never pick up a thing. Whether or not you are predisposed to athlete's foot depends on a combination of luck plus the general effectiveness of your personal immune system. This is a combination whose effectiveness cannot be accurately forecasted.

Perhaps you've also wondered how exactly to diagnose athlete's foot. This is simple, because the condition always has a highly individual symptom. If you have a white, macerated area with cracking skin located between the fourth and fifth toes of your foot, then you've got athlete's foot. If you *don't* have that symptom, then whatever it is on your foot, it's probably not a fungus. If you have rashes on the tops of your toes, it's probably either eczema or an allergic reaction to your own shoes. Antifungal medicines of the sort described below will only make it worse. The most soothing thing you can do for foot rashes is treat them with zinc oxide paste. If they're really bothersome, your doctor may prescribe an antiinflammatory steroid cream.

However, if you've got the maceration and cracking between the fourth and fifth toes, then it's a good bet you've got a fungus. Many people wonder if they could have prevented the infection. Keeping the feet dry with daily applications of talc or cornstarch powders is the best prevention—but it only helps to a degree. Fungi don't thrive in dry environments. But if you have a predisposition to fungal infections, then you're just going to have a high risk of getting them.

The big news in antifungal foot therapy is the general availability of a chemical called tolnaftate. This is a superlatively effective antifungal, which for years was available with a prescription only. Today you can buy it in a number of OTC products. Among them, my top recommendation goes (primarily because of its reasonable price) to AFTATE ANTIFUNGAL, which comes in powder, spray powder, spray liquid, and gel forms. This is unquestionably the best commercial athlete's-foot preparation on the market.

Equally effective, although more expensive, is TINACTIN. This, too, is based on tolnaftate, and it comes in powder, spray powder, and cream forms.

Athlete's foot has traditionally been a problem in armies, doubtless due to wet feet and insufficient foot hygiene. The United States Army experimented for years before finally settling on a chemical called "undecylenic acid" as its favored antifungal agent. This chemical is contained in numerous traditional athlete's-foot medications, all of which predate the OTC availability of tolnaftate.

The following undecylenic-acid preparations all work, but I don't consider them as effective as those made with tolnaftate.

DESENEX (in powder, spray powder, ointment, and soap forms)

QUINSANA PLUS MEDICATED FOOT POWDER

SCHOLL FOOT POWDER SPRAY

CALLUSES

GILLETTE FOOT GUARD ANTIFUNGAL FOOT DEODORANT MEDICATED FOOT CARE

NP 27 SPRAY POWDER (Norwich Products)

Before undecylenic acid was available, the traditional approach to fungal infections on the feet was to peel them off with salicylic acid. A few preparations of this sort still remain on the market. DR. SCHOLL'S SOLVEX ATHLETE'S FOOT POWDER (not to be confused with his spray, pump, or spray powder) is one, as is DR. SCHOLL'S SOLVEX ATHLETE'S FOOT OINTMENT. These are old-fashioned cures that aren't nearly as effective as undecylenic acid or tolnaftate.

Scholl makes a myriad of similar-sounding foot remedies, which, for the most part, are quite good. However, I would caution you *against* DR. SCHOLL'S SOLVEX ATHLETE'S FOOT SPRAY, SPRAY POWDER, and PUMP SPRAY. These products contain benzocaine, a soothing local pain killer that also happens to be a potent allergen. I don't think this ingredient is necessary in antifungal therapy, and there's no reason to expose yourself to any known allergen unless there's a real reason.

Calluses

Calluses are caused by a repeated physical trauma on the same spot. In effect, a callus is the body's attempt to protect itself by thickening the skin where the trauma occurs.

The problem with calluses on the feet is that they often make walking uncomfortable. This is especially true when calluses are left unattended and allowed to become too large. Usually a callus is the direct result of lousy (meaning tight or ill-fitting) shoes. Recurrent or particularly painful calluses may require a visit to a podiatrist or different shoes, or both.

If your calluses only cause minimum discomfort, you can easily treat them at home. Don't try to whittle at them as if they were a wood carving. Instead, go out and buy a BUF PUF. This is an abrasive, nonmedicated, polyester sponge sold in drugstores and recommended elsewhere in this book for epiabrasion. Here I want to recommend it for preventing and controlling calluses on the feet. Keeping a Buf Puf in the shower and using it daily to wash your feet makes excellent sense. Its abrasive action keeps potential calluses from building up.

I think daily use of the Buf Puf is wiser than waiting for the calluses to become uncomfortable. Some people let them go to that point, then try to correct the damage with a medicated foot bath. CORN-O-CIDE MEDICATED FOOT BATH is a popular one. Besides cooling menthol and soothing sodium carbonate, it contains methyl salicylate to soften the calluses and make them easier to scrape down. But if your feet are callus prone, it seems much more sensible to me to institute a daily cleansing regimen with a Buf Puf; then you'll never have a callus that gets out of control.

PRODUCTS FOR THE FEET

Do You Suffer From Ingrown Toenails?

Not many people do, but that's small comfort if *you've* got one. How do they get ingrown? It's no mystery, really. Toenails often grow into surrounding flesh when they are incorrectly cut. Cut your toenails straight across; don't try and trim them down the sides toward the cuticle. If you haven't followed this advice, and an ingrown nail has caused a corner of your toe to swell and hurt, try treating the area with BACITRACIN, an OTC antibacterial cream. Bacitracin is great for speeding the departure of minor infections, which makes ingrown toenails so uncomfortable. Of course, if the pain is extreme, see a doctor.

CHAPTER 12

Wart Remedies

Every doctor has a wart story, and every mother has a unique (and usually startling) cure for warts. Wart stories make regular appearances in what's called the *Shoch Letter,* a professional dermatological monthly distributed to the trade by the American Academy of Dermatology. The *Shoch Letter* consists entirely of anecdotes about some of the wild inspirations that (much to everyone's surprise) actually effect a cure. Lately, I've read of warts being cleared up by applications of formalin (an embalming substance) and of lemon juice, by injections of chopped-up warts, and smallpox vaccinations. Unfortunately, none of these remedies seems to work on everybody.

In every single grossly swollen cell of a wart, there is at least one wart virus. The key to removing the wart is to kill the viruses. And interestingly, *the* most deadly and effective agent against these viruses is your own personal immunology—your body's ability to produce antibodies. If warts are left alone and not assaulted by electric needles, acids, fingernails, razor blades and what have you, they will, in ninety-five cases out of a hundred, be destroyed naturally by your own body.

People take their warts to doctors for a variety of reasons. For one thing, warts can be painful. For another, American patients like action; they don't want to hear how warts will just go away by themselves. And warts can also be frightening; to look at a lump on your body is to see the word "tumor" blaze across the mind. Warts may come in a dazzling variety of sizes and shapes (not to mention locations), but they are usually quite benign. Perhaps what most justifies a visit to the doctor is having a wart appear somewhere that is either embarrassing (the tip of your nose or the end of your forefinger) or painful or prone to irritation (as, for example, on the sole of the foot or in the genital region).

Unless you have one of these cases, you can easily speed the departure of your warts right at home with the help of simple nonprescription drugstore items. Because of the high incidence of spontaneous improvement, however, it is not easy to evaluate the efficacy of individual wart remedies. Wart removal is an area of medicine in which the placebo effect is considerable; bear in mind that

WART REMEDIES

your own immunology is what eventually kills the virus. This explains to some extent the long tradition of nostrums—paint them green, sleep with a bat wing under your pillow, wish them away—that has grown up around warts.

Psychology can often play a positive role in wart therapy, which brings to mind a story about a very talented dermatologist I once knew. Much of his practice was with children, who as a group are very susceptible to warts. He would, in effect, implant a strong suggestion in the kids' minds by telling them he had a "magic wart medicine" that would make the warts disappear in seven days. It hardly mattered what was in the medicine—sometimes it was just calamine lotion—but the kids' suggestibility worked wonders.

Don't think that mental set is a critical factor only among children. Studies have shown that if cold viruses are sprayed up the noses of a random sample of adults, those who are unhappy and depressed will be much more likely to get a cold. Why? Because state of mind has a direct correlation to the physical ability to produce antibodies.

The answer to the question, "Are warts catching?" rests in large part on one's susceptibility. Both disposition and suggestibility play a large part in this. If your personal immunology is not functioning well, you'll be as liable to succumb to wart viruses as to cold viruses. If it is, you won't. Some teachers who deal with kids all day catch warts. I examine and come in contact with warts every week. I've only had one in my life, and I am not at all certain it was picked up from a patient.

In our culture, most wart sufferers become obsessed with prompt removal. But the latest medical thinking indicates that vigorous attack on warts *does not* hasten their departure. In other words, those who burn, pick, freeze, or shave warts are mistaken if they think these measures are making the wart go away any faster than simply leaving it alone. Often these approaches give only the illusion of hastening wart removal. My own wart was right on the tip of my finger—a bad spot for a wart, especially for a doctor. First I had it burned off with an electric needle; it came back. Next, I had it frozen with liquid nitrogen; it came back again. After that, I began to shave it down every day. After eight weeks, it finally left me. In retrospect, I think all my efforts were a waste. What's worse, although the methods of removal aren't so painful while in process, the affected area becomes uncomfortable later on. I now believe I should have just left my wart alone under a Band-Aid.

Commercial wart remedies all work pretty much alike. They contain an ingredient to soften the affected skin (usually salicylic acid) and various additives to insure that the active ingredient will adhere to the warty area. It is believed that the softening action itself somehow stimulates the body's immune reaction. In other words, wart remedies don't kill wart viruses, but rather goad the body into doing it. Possibly these remedies encourage a faster antibody attack on wart viruses, but proof of this is elusive.

It's thought, too, that if you eradicate the "mother wart" (in cases of multiple warts, the "mother" is the first that appeared), the others will go away more quickly. Finding the mother is not always easy. It is not necessarily the biggest, and there are wart sufferers who host literally hundreds of warts. I once had a patient with approximately five hundred warts on his fingers. He came to me for four successive visits, and each time I picked one large single wart to attack with either liquid nitrogen or an electric needle. On the fourth visit, I apparently hit the mother, because within two weeks they suddenly all went away!

May you be spared five hundred warts on your fingers. If you develop a few (or even one) I recommend that you go to a drugstore and purchase a 40% salicylic acid plaster. A company named Duke makes a good one, but other concerns manufacture equally effective 40% plasters.

The "plaster" is merely an adhesive-backed foam-rubber pad permeated with salicylic acid. You cut it out with scissors to cover your wart, being sure not to let it overlap the unaffected skin by more than a quarter inch. The plaster is particularly recommended for warts on the fingers and feet. The latter are called "plantar" warts; the word derives from the *plan*tar (or bottom) of the *tar*sus bone (of your foot). The plaster is left on for a week, after which the macerated skin that develops beneath it is scraped away with any handy clean (not necessarily sterile) instrument—a small knife, manicure implement, razor blade, or whatever. Don't be concerned if there is a little bleeding; that's normal. The process should be repeated at least once more, after which you may want to give the area a rest to see if the wart is really gone. If not, repeat the treatment weekly until it is. Most warts respond within eight weeks.

If you suffer repeatedly from plantar warts, it may be a result either of the way you walk or the shoes you wear. You may be inflicting a repetitive trauma on the feet, which can give the wart virus a chance to establish itself. Remember, too, that your body hosts many microorganisms that lie dormant. It's possible to have a wart virus in your system without having a wart. When a wart does appear, it can very well be a result of physical trauma, as opposed to contact with a wart carrier. If plantar warts are driving you crazy and you cannot get relief from 40% salicylic acid plasters, I recommend that you consider seeing an orthopedist.

The best-selling OTC wart remedy is COMPOUND W, a household treatment that legions of Americans swear by. It comes in a little bottle with a glass rod applicator attached to the cap. You apply drops of the medicine twice daily for about a week, scrubbing the area with a brush or washcloth before each application. Compound W is salicylic acid, plus acetic acid, menthol, camphor (for a cooling feeling), and castor oil. I think it's an excellent product; it's even guaranteed to work or your money back.

VERGO is a gentler OTC wart product whose active skin-softening ingredient is a substance they call pancin (a formulation of calcium pantothenate, ascorbic acid, and starch). Vergo is applied daily, then sealed under a Band-Aid to encourage absorption (just like a plaster). It's recommended mainly for children.

WART REMEDIES

Interestingly, covering a wart with a Band-Aid is sometimes all the treatment that's needed. This phenomenon is not fully understood, but it is a medically observable fact. I must caution that if additional warts begin to appear while you're treating yourself with any of the medicines above, it is *not* the fault of the medicine. Wart remedies simply have no effect on wart viruses. If warts begin to proliferate, it's spontaneous. The visible wart is a symptom, not the cause of the virus.

If you visit a doctor for plantar or venereal warts (these are simply warts in the genital or anal region), he may tell you to get one of the following three prescription preparations: DUOFILM is a popular product similar to Compound W, just stronger. CANTHARONE is interesting stuff. Its active ingredient is obtained from a secretion of the blister beetle. It works a little like liquid nitrogen; application causes the skin to blister, after which the wart viruses are literally floated out of the affected region by the fluid that collects and eventually drains away. Finally, there's VER-VAR, a potent preparation whose main ingredient is called podophyllin. Ver-var destroys not only warts, but also senile and seborrheic keratoses (crusty lesions that affect the skin of old people) as well as a host of benign skin tumors. It is often the preferred treatment for venereal warts.

CHAPTER 13

Sun Care Products

Suntans are attractive, but getting them can be dangerous because certain of the sun's tanning rays can harm the skin—both in the short and long run.

The rays that cause tanning are called "ultraviolet" (uv). uv rays have varying wave lengths; some don't hurt the skin; others do. The damaging rays cause harm first by precipitating sunburn. (Let me interject that, contrary to many people's belief, it is *not* necessary to get burned before you get tanned. Customary, yes; necessary, no.) What happens with a sunburn is that the damaging rays inflame the skin, while at the same time causing close-to-the-surface blood vessels to dilate. These two phenomena cause redness. Blood vessel dilation—called "vasodilatation"—has another critical effect: it makes the blood vessel walls leak. They leak irritating toxins and blood serum that would otherwise remain in the bloodstream away from the skin. The presence of toxins (impurities that would otherwise be filtered from the blood by the liver, kidneys, etc.) causes pain in the skin tissue. The serum causes the tissues to swell and blister. Even if the blisters are "subclinical" (meaning not easy to see with the naked eye) they still behave like blisters, which means that, once the swelling goes down, the top layer of skin will peel off. That is why sunburns peel.

Accumulated years of sun exposure can cause problems far more serious than sunburn. Both premature aging and skin cancer are directly linked to cumulative unprotected exposure to damaging uv rays. It may take decades, but these uv rays can eventually disrupt the delicate molecular balance of healthy, growing skin cells. And when that balance is upset, unsightly lesions or cancerous cell proliferation can result. "Elastin," the protein structures that give skin its tone, can also be gradually destroyed by the sun. Premature sagging and drooping of the flesh result.

A suntan is actually the body's own means of protecting itself from the damaging sun rays. Skin that's tanned has a more thorough distribution of the pigmenting substance called melanin, which is contained in every cell. The melanin, when distributed throughout the skin cells, screens out most of the damaging rays

SUN CARE PRODUCTS

and inhibits their effect on elastin structures and molecular processes within each cell.

To understand more clearly how a tan occurs, consider a skin cell like a glass of milk with a glob of chocolate syrup on the bottom. As long as the glass remains unstirred, the milk will appear predominantly white and the syrup will be limited to the bottom of the glass. Similarly, a skin cell that hasn't been exposed to much sunlight will remain relatively unpigmented since the melanin it contains will naturally keep to itself. But once you lie down by the pool and start to bake, the sun's UV rays trigger an automatic melanin disbursement within the cells of the sun-exposed skin. This is analogous to stirring the glass of milk. Just as it will start to turn brown from the chocolate, so the skin cells will begin to color from the disbursed melanin. Result: a tan. The longer you expose your skin to UV sun rays, the more thorough this disbursement will be, causing an increasingly darker tan. UV exposure also stimulates the production of additional melanin, and, if exposure continues, this will in turn be distributed throughout each cell, making the tan darker still.

It's interesting to note that people with naturally black or darkly pigmented skin have an inherited protection against UV rays. Skin is practically identical among the races of man, save for the degree of melanin distribution. Black people, for example, often don't have any more melanin per cell than white people. It's just distributed more thoroughly from birth. Which is why black people rarely suffer from skin cancer or sun-related loss of skin tone.

Sunscreens

"Sunscreens"—the proper term for all the tanning lotions, gels, foams, oils, and creams on the market today—screen out most (not all) damaging UV rays. People who don't spend their lives in the sun need these products for the first few days of sun exposure *only*. This is a key point, since many vacationers think they have to keep using their suntan stuff all vacation long. Not so. You need a sunscreen only until you develop enough of a tan so that your body can do its own UV screening without getting sunburned.

People who spend their lives in the sun—farmers, tennis pros, ski instructors, construction workers, etc.—*do,* however, need sunscreen protection all the time. That's because suntans, like sunscreens, provide only *partial* protection against damaging UV rays. The damage to elastin and cellular organization is slow and cumulative, so, if you spend your life in the sun, you need the extra protection of the sunscreen even if you have a good, dark tan.

The undisputed best sunscreen agent available at present is called "Paba," which stands for para-amino-benzoid acid. There are several Paba substitutes, most of which predate the development of Paba itself, but none is nearly as effective as Paba in screening out damaging UV rays.

Because of Paba's effectiveness, it's recently been included in the formulas of some products that have been around for many years. This augmentation has not always made the products more effective. Because of its chemical nature, Paba works best in an alcohol base. It does not work very well at all in many of the oily formulas to which it's recently been added. Let me add that Paba works best in low concentrations, usually in no more than a 5% solution. Interestingly, a product that is more than 5% Paba actually provides *less* sunscreen protection than a 5% concentration.

Medically speaking, whether or not a suntan product "works well" is simply a function of whether or not it contains Paba and alcohol. Anything else in the formula is mere window dressing. Users of home-mixed combos of mineral oil and iodine take note. There is *no* reason to spread oil or grease on the skin while sunning. Oily substances in *no* way affect UV rays or the reaction of skin-cell melanin. They neither protect nor promote tanning. They are only a vehicle for Paba, and, as stated earlier, oil makes a rather bad vehicle, since Paba works vastly better in an alcohol base.

The four products below are the best sunscreens you can get. Each contains Paba in a predominantly alcohol base, and each will amply protect the skin during the critical first days of sun exposure.

> PRESUN 5% PABA GEL (by Westwood Pharmaceuticals)
>
> PABANOL (by Paul B. Elder Co.)
>
> PABAGEL PURE PABA SUNSCREEN GEL (by Owen Labs)
>
> PABAFILM SUNSCREEN GEL (by Owen Labs)

I also recommend a Paba lipstick that may protect the lips from herpes eruptions (fever blisters), which sometimes seem to be provoked by sun exposure. It's called RV PABA LIPSTICK, and it's made from a combination of Paba and red petrolatum, an old-fashioned, mildly effective sunscreen that's a cousin to Vaseline.

Paba products must all be thoroughly and carefully applied lest you miss a spot. (Application is not made easier by most of the products being clear.) The manufacturers recommend that you apply their products from thirty minutes to an hour before sun exposure. I think that as long as they're dry by the time you go out in the sun, you'll be O. K. Paba washes off in water, so you must scrupulously reapply it after you swim or if you're perspiring freely. Care should be taken when using Paba around synthetic fabrics. It causes yellow stains on certain man-made fibers, so be careful if you're wearing a white synthetic-fiber bathing suit.

Paba is also contained in the products on the list below, but since all these have oil-based formulas, the Paba protection is diminished accordingly.

> ALMAY SEMI-FILTER SUN LOTION, ALMAY FULL-FILTER SUN LOTION, and ALMAY DEEP TANNING OIL (by Almay, Inc.)

SUN CARE PRODUCTS

SUPER SHADE SUNBLOCKING LOTION BY COPPERTONE (by Plough, Inc.)

BAIN DE SOLEIL SUPER FILTER SUNTAN LOTION and BAIN DE SOLEIL SUNTAN LOTION (by Lanvin-Charles of the Ritz)

TROPICAL DELUXE FORMULA DARK TANNING OIL (by Lanvin-Charles of the Ritz)

SEA & SKI SUNTAN LOTION (by Sea & Ski Corp.; contains a close chemical cousin of Paba)

ECLIPSE SUNSCREEN LOTION (by Herbert Labs)

APOLLO SUN FOR A SAFE, DARK TAN (by Apollo Sun Ltd.)

ALMAY SUN BLOC GEL, ALMAY DEEP TANNING CREAM, and ALMAY SEMI-FILTER SUN CREME (by Almay, Inc.)

BAIN DE SOLEIL WHITE NON-OILY SUNTAN CREME, BAIN DE SOLEIL SUNTAN CREME, and BAIN DE SOLEIL SUNTAN FOAM (by Lanvin-Charles of the Ritz)

It's interesting to note that, although the above list contains products that would seem to perform very different functions (dark tanning oils as opposed to sun blocks), they all perform in approximately the *same* manner. Every one contains oils—including the ones that claim to be nonoily—that have no effect whatsoever on tanning, plus Paba that screens damaging UV rays, albeit less effectively than it would in an alcohol base.

I can't think why the makers of certain of the above products toss around the term "sun block" (or "bloc," if you will) so casually. Paba, for all its effectiveness, is hardly a sunblock. That term is applied to substances that screen out *all* the rays of the sun, and it's for people who don't want any tan at all. Zinc oxide paste, the white, tacky stuff that lifeguards wear on their noses, is the prototype sun block. When applied to the skin, this paste will not permit a single ray to penetrate. Of course, it can also make you look like a clown. A better idea for people who need this level of protection is Å-FIL CREAM, described by its makers (Texas Pharmaceuticals) as "the sunscreen [sic] that went to the moon with NASA." Å-Fil contains titanium dioxide, a paste similar to zinc oxide, in a color-tinted cream base. I recommend it highly for people whose skin cannot tolerate any sun exposure at all, either due to a burn or to general sensitivity. Just remember that you won't get *any* tan with a sun block.

As for the "deep tanning" claims of some of the above products, well, oils *don't* tan you deeper. Adding Paba to the oil simply provides a measure of sunscreen protection that will neither inhibit nor encourage your rate of tanning. As a group, these products are very misleadingly labeled.

Paba may be the best, but it is by no means the only sunscreen ingredient on the market. All the Paba substitutes, however, have an approximately equal level of effectiveness—which is way below that of Paba. One of these substitutes is called "homosalate," and it's the active ingredient in perhaps the most popular suntan family of them all—COPPERTONE. Homosalate was around for years before Paba, and it does provide moderate—albeit less effective—sunscreen protection. Coppertone is still clinging to its homosalate formulas, which is why I can't give a very high recommendation to either their Suntan Lotion, Suntan Oil, or Tanning Butter.

In many northern latitudes, the summer sun is rather weak, and many sunbathers don't notice Coppertone's lack of Paba. Unfortunately, Coppertone is frequently the only product you can buy in tropical resorts. And it's exactly in these places that visitors desperately need Paba protection. This is why you're well advised to buy Paba sunscreens *before* you leave for a destination outside the United States.

An update on Coppertone: even they've finally given in to the Paba rage and included it in their SUPER SHADE SUNBLOCKING LOTION mentioned earlier. Of course this product is in no way a sun block, since it will allow you to tan. One wonders if some diehard homosalate fan misleadingly dubbed it a "block" in a bit of envy.

Besides homosalate, there are other sunscreens, such as padimate (contained in SUNGUARD LOTION, and SEA & SKI GOLDEN TAN); cinoxate (found in SUNDARE SUNSCREEN CREAMY LOTION, and SUNDARE SUNSCREEN CLEAR LOTION); dimethyl amino benzoate (in SEA & SKI DARK TANNING OIL); red petrolatum (found in RVP WIDE-SPECTRUM SUNSCREEN); and cinnamate (contained in MOON DROPS BRONZE LUSTRE). None of these chemicals is recommended over any other, and they are all approximately as effective as homosalate. None can hold a candle to Paba when it comes to screening out damaging UV rays.

Another sun care product that's quite popular is a gel derived from the tropical Aloe Vera plant. Products with Aloe are creamy and good smelling, but does Aloe either moisturize or protect the skin from the sun's burning rays? I'm afraid there is no evidence that it does. A company called Aloe Creme Labs makes several Aloe products, among them ALO FASHION TAN SUNTAN MOISTURIZER (whose ingredients include Aloe Vera gel, homosalate, mineral oil, and lanolin), ALO SUPER RICH TAN (with Aloe Vera gel, mineral oil, cocoa butter, and Paba), and ALO SUN BLOCK LOTION (a misleadingly named concoction of Aloe Vera gel, Paba, cocoa butter, lanolin, and moisture-holding urea). The products that contain Paba do offer some sunscreen protection. However, that is seriously diminished by the high oil content of the formulas. ALO FASHION TAN SUNTAN MOISTURIZER without Paba smells and feels great, but it does nothing at all either to promote a good tan or to prevent peeling, and the homosalate content affords minimal sunscreen protection. The manufacturer makes much of Aloe's supposed ability to moisturize, but actually there isn't much you can do to seal in moisture while you're

SUN CARE PRODUCTS

out in the sun. The way to prevent après-sun dryness is by hydration and by applying a water-sealing moisturizer *after* sun exposure. More about that later in this chapter.

Two other Aloe products, made by Lauderdale Cosmetics, are marketed under the not-very-subtle names of FOREPLAY SUNTAN OIL and FOREPLAY SUNTAN LOTION. The former contains Aloe, coconut oil, and Vitamin E, and it's hard to imagine a group of ingredients less related to tanning and sunscreen protection. The lotion form is the same stuff minus the coconut oil, and it's equally ineffective. The name is a pun on the product's supposed usefulness "wherever there's outdoor action."

Finally, I must mention those products that "tan" you whether or not you even go out in the sun. The white chemical powder responsible for this miracle is called dihydroxy acetone. It's a coal-tar derivative with no known toxicity. All it does is color skin orangey brown without the aid of sunlight. QT LOTION and QT FOAM (both by Plough, Inc.) are dihydroxy acetone preparations that include the sunscreen homosalate. INDOOR/OUTDOOR TANNING LOTION (by Sea & Ski Corp.) is another dihydroxy acetone product with padimate instead of homosalate. None of these products is a superior sunscreen because of the absence of Paba in their formulas. Each, however, will safely impart an artificial color to supplement whatever tan you may acquire. The more natural sun you get, the less phony the dihydroxy acetone coloring will look. There are also people whose natural coloration complements the otherwise artificial-looking orangey brown in a way that makes it look natural. I don't really recommend these products, because I prefer the look of natural tans. However, they are safe and they do work.

The Best Ways to Tan Safely

If you're heading for a vacation in the tropics and you haven't been in the sun for months (or longer), do the following: on the first day out, spend no more than two minutes walking around in the sun without any sunscreen. Then go into the shade and apply one of the Paba and alcohol sunscreens recommended at the beginning of this chapter and let it dry. These sunscreens are truly amazing. If you apply them to all sun-exposed parts of the body and keep reapplying when necessary, you simply will not get a sunburn—even on a blazing tropical Caribbean beach. Depending on the progress of your tan, you can diminish the amount of Paba sunscreen you use, until finally you can just go out in the sun with no sunscreen protection at all. The point at which you can dispense with the sunscreen varies with the individual, but it is no mystery. Your body will tell you when you're tanned enough to skip the Paba.

If you're vacationing or summering in a northern latitude where the sun isn't strong, Paba still provides the best short-term antisunburn protection as well as long-term protection from damaging UV rays. Remember, the long-term damage is slow and cumulative. Today you may be in love with a sunscreen that contains no Paba, but thirty years from now you may deeply regret not having given your skin Paba protection over the years. Since the other sunscreen agents are all weaker than Paba, they always present a greater chance of sunburn as well as cellular damage.

If you spend your working life in the sunshine, you definitely should make Paba a part of that life. It will help protect you against the possibility of skin cancer as well as premature aging. By all means use it every day, especially on the face, neck, hands, arms, or anywhere else that gets frequent sun exposure.

Aftersun Moisturizers

Many people mistakenly think that by applying oils to the skin after sunning, they will prevent peeling. First of all, oils in themselves do not moisturize the skin, they only retard the evaporation of moisture that's already in the skin. And even proper moisturization—meaning hydration followed by application of an oily moisturizer—won't have any effect on peeling if you've allowed yourself to get a sunburn. Remember that the vasodilatation from sunburn allows blood serum to seep into the skin and cause swelling and subclinical blistering. If you're bright red after a day of sun, you'd better believe that you have at least some subclinical blistering. That means that some amount of peeling is inevitable, no matter how much aftersun oil you apply.

If you don't want to peel, don't let yourself get burned. Trying to stop peeling by applying oils in the evening is really closing the barn door after the horse is long gone. And don't confuse the peeling that follows sunburn with dry skin. They are unrelated.

Most of the time, suntan candidates swim, golf, and play tennis in summery and usually humid climates. Just the humidity in the air is frequently enough to prevent the dryness that might otherwise result from daylong exposure to dehydrating water and sunshine. If you're vacationing in a desert climate, however, you probably will need to moisturize your skin at the end of the day—*not* to prevent peeling, but just to avoid the uncomfortable tautness and/or prickly sensation of dry skin. Moisturize the same way you do on a normal day without sun exposure. Hydrate the skin by bathing in lukewarm water (hot water opens the pores too much and encourages afterbath dehydration), pat dry, and apply your favorite moisturizer. This can be any preparation whose oily base helps slow the evaporation of moisture from the surface of the skin. Or it can be a product like AQUACARE that contains "urea," an aquaphilic chemical that attracts and holds moisture.

Most aftersun moisturizers imply that they will help you keep a tan longer. But if you read the label claims closely, you'll discover that they never quite say so in so many words. Instead they purport to "aid in retention" of your tan, or "help keep you glowing," or "give your tan a silkier, softer look," and so on. The people who write these claims are equivocating because they know

SUN CARE PRODUCTS

very well that mineral oil, lanolin, Aloe, Vitamin E, or whatever else aftersun products contain, really has *no* effect on either peeling or tanning.

Most aftersun moisturizers are at least as good as ordinary moisturizers. I personally like the feel and smell of APRÈS LE SOLEIL (by Lanvin-Charles of the Ritz), ALO AFTER TAN (by Aloe Creme Labs, Inc.), and TAN CARE BY COPPERTONE (by Plough, Inc.). However, don't expect these or similar products to do more than ordinary moisturizers. They contain no ingredient that can make tans last longer. The way to do that is, again, not to burn.

Sunburn Remedies

Before we talk about remedies, let me say a few words about prevention. The first and foremost means of preventing sunburn, of course, is use of a Paba sunscreen. But besides Paba, you should know about the many common substances that are "photosensitizing"—which cause adverse skin reactions in the presence of sunlight. By themselves, these photosensitizing substances are relatively harmless. But if you take, use, eat, or apply any one of them before or during sun exposure, you dramatically increase your chances of getting a bad sunburn.

Common Photosensitizing Substances

    Birth control pills

    Water pills

    Anticonvulsive medicines

    Oral antidiabetic medicines

    Lemon juice or essences (applied topically)

    Lime juice or essences (applied topically)

    Deodorant soaps

    Perfumes or colognes (with oil of bergamot)

    Artificially sweetened soft drinks

If you do get a burn, how do you treat it? First, stay completely out of the sun. Next, take a cool, short bath. If any areas are particularly painful, apply the soothing compress described back in the Introduction. Aspirin seems to help relieve sunburn pain, too. Be patient; sunburns usually peak in forty-eight hours. And finally, apply a pain-killing sunburn remedy of the sort described below.

Most sunburn remedies contain the topical anesthetic benzocaine—or, occasionally, a close chemical relative of it. This substance—as well as its chemical relations—soothes pain by deadening surface nerve endings. Benzocaine products also contain oils that lubricate burned tissue and help prevent dryness by sealing in moisture. Unfortunately, many people are allergic to benzocaine. For them, applying this type of sunburn pain killer will actually provoke a painful rash on top of the sunburn. If any benzocaine product does this to you, discontinue its use immediately, bathe the affected area in cool water, and apply the antiinflammatory compress referred to earlier. There's no sense switching to any of the other benzocaine products, because if you're allergic to one, you'll have the same reaction to others.

I'm glad to report that the overwhelming majority of people will have no problems at all with benzocaine products. The following is a list of my favorites:

> SOLARCAINE LOTION and SOLARCAINE SPRAY (by Plough, Inc.)
>
> KIP FIRST AID SPRAY and KIP SUNBURN LOTION (by Kip, Inc.)
>
> NUPERCAINAL PAIN RELIEF LOTION and NUPERCAINAL PAIN RELIEF CREAM (by Ciba Pharmaceutical Co.)

If you can't use a benzocaine (or dibucaine, or anything else that ends with "-caine") remedy due to allergic reaction, there are several soothing second choices. REGULAR NOXZEMA SKIN CREAM (by Noxell), won't deaden pain, but it will cool and lubricate. You might also try VASELINE CAMPHOR ICE SKIN BALM, (by Chesebrough-Pond's, Inc.) whose camphor content feels cooling and acts as a mild topical anesthetic. CALADRYL LOTION (by Parke-Davis) contains a topical anesthetic called benadryl, and, even though this product is often thought to be solely against poison ivy, it's actually excellent in deadening sunburn pain. Finally, I recommend SEA BREEZE ANTISEPTIC FOR THE SKIN (by Sea Breeze Labs, Inc.) which contains cooling camphor and alcohol plus soothing oil of clove. Many of my patients particularly like the feel and smell of this product, and I pass their recommendation along to you.

CHAPTER 14

Masks

Masks are substances applied to the face with a brush or the fingers, allowed to dry, and removed either with water or peeled away with the fingers. Masks are purely for fun. They won't make you beautiful or affect your complexion in any but the most temporary way. But even if they don't do much for your skin (this in spite of manufacturers' claims) they usually smell great, feel tingly, cleanse the skin (to a certain minimal degree) of surface debris and dead skin cells, and (like astringents) leave the pores temporarily tightened.

Masks have been a favorite cosmetic for as long as there have been cosmetics. Perhaps this historic popularity stems from the mask as a symbol of transformation. Surely the attractive scent and packaging of today's mask products increase their appeal. And they're so benign that most people can use them as often as they choose.

Medically speaking, the purpose of using a mask is "epiabrasion." This is a concept I've already discussed. To recapitulate briefly, epiabrasion is the medical name for mild abrasion (call it gentle scrubbing, if you will) of the epidermis, or top layers of the skin. Epiabrasion improves the appearance by stimulating the circulation and giving the complexion a rosier glow; lowering the incidence of acne by effectively removing excess oil and incipient oil plugs; improving the health of the skin by promoting a more efficient skin-cell turnover rate; and reducing the appearance of wrinkles by puffing them up by causing a minimal and harmless amount of subcutaneous fluid collection.

Actually, the best way to epiabrade is not with a mask. To get the full benefits described above, use a BUF PUF, a synthetic sponge sold in drugstores and used mostly in teenage acne therapy. The next best way to epiabrade is simply by scrubbing the face with a washcloth—being careful, of course, not to rub yourself raw. Masks are the mildest form of epiabrasion, since they involve no scrubbing. They remove unwanted surface material simply by taking it along with them when they're removed. This method is obviously a much less thorough means of cleansing and stimulating the skin than use of either the Buf Puf or a washcloth.

Masks, however, are decidedly more fun. And almost every mask on the market brings about noticeable tightening and temporary toning of the skin, is easy to apply and remove, causes no discomfort or irritation.

I think the peel-off masks are better than the rinse-off varieties, because they most enhance the epiabrasive effect. My favorite is Max Factor's BLUE MASK, a product with numerous good points. It's applied with a well-designed brush applicator (instead of messy fingers), and, when it dries (unfortunately, not for forty minutes), you can pinpoint the exact location of problem dry and oily areas. For diagnostic purposes, the mask is applied to an unwashed face. When it's removed—you peel it down from the forehead—skin flakes will indicate problem dry areas, shiny patches will show the boundaries of your overly oily areas, and smooth and dull patches will show exactly where you're normal. In effect, you'll be getting a detailed map of your face that can help you decide how to treat and maintain it. The activity of facial oil glands and oiliness of the skin vary considerably from one section of the face to another. The big value of the Blue Mask is that it can show you exactly where to do what. If, however, you're using the mask purely for its epiabrasive, skin-toning, and pore-tightening effects, you must wash the face well before application. In that case, you won't get the facial oil profile described above.

Other good peel-off masks include Helena Rubinstein's BRUSH-ON PEEL-OFF MASK (which comes with very good commonsensical directions as well as a brush applicator; time required is ten minutes); Etherea's FRESH SKIN (seductively scented and packaged, if a little expensive; time required is fifteen minutes); Helena Rubinstein's BIO-CLEAR (slightly drying for blemish control); and Coty's PEEL AWAY MASK.

Alternatively, you can make a very good peeling mask at home with an egg white for a fraction of the cost of a prepared product. Use ¼ teaspoon flowers of sulphur (a drugstore item for removing skin oil), ¼ teaspoon alum (also a drugstore item, for tightening the pores), and the white of one egg. Mix well with a fork in a small bowl, apply with the fingers, and peel off when dry. The commercially prepared products are simply fancy substitutes for this simple recipe. In fairness, however, I must note that they are easier to apply and more cosmetically attractive.

Masks that aren't peeled off are rinsed away, and there are many more of this type available. My favorite is SEBA-NIL CLEANSING MASK, widely available and quite effective as a prophylactic for acne-prone skin. Seba-Nil contains bentonite and alcohol, and so can be overly drying to some skins. It's also a little hard to wash off. Still, as masks go, it's excellent for removing surface oils, dead skin cells, and dirt.

Other good, reasonably priced rinse-off masks include:

MEDICATED MASQUE (by Bonne Bell)

QUEEN HELENE MINT JULEP MASQUE (by Para Labs)

MASKS

SUDDEN BEAUTY COUNTRY AIR MASK (by Whitehall Labs)

MASQUE FRAPPÉ (by Dorothy Gray)

Many other masks of the rinse-off type are based on mud or clay. These include products like Scandia's STIMULUS NATURAL CLAY MASQUE, Etherea's ACTIVE MUD MASQUE, and Princess Marcella Borghese's CLAY MASQUE. For some reason clay-based masks often cost more. Is it because only special, exotic clays can "remove all traces of surface impurities," or "tighten and firm" the skin, or "vacuum clean away excess oil, soil and cellular debris?" No, it's not. If you go to a hobby store, purchase normal modeling clay, mix it at home with water, and spread it over your face, you will obtain exactly the same cleansing effect. The only things you'll sacrifice are a stylish package, an attractive scent, and a few needless ingredients.

I won't bother knocking the high-priced beauty masks of Clinique, Chanel, Charles of the Ritz, Orlane, Lancôme, or anyone else. If their color, consistency, and smell delight you, by all means use them. They will certainly work as well as any of my recommendations. Just don't expect a facial mask—*any* facial mask—to have any lasting effect whatsoever on your skin's moisture content, pore size, degree of cleanliness, surface, texture, or anything else, because masks are just for fun.

What of "medicated" masks and those with "special moisturizers"? Phooey! The "medicines" are typically unspectacular protein additives that have nothing to do with epiabrasion. And expecting to moisturize your face with a mask is to ignore completely the cardinal rule of moisturization: first hydrate the skin, then lock the moisture in with a moisturizer.

Zizmor's Rubifactant Mask

For: A stimulating do-it-yourself "mini-peel" to temporarily enhance the rosiness of the complexion and make wrinkles less noticeable

How it works: By the use of natural "rubifactants"—substances that stimulate the skin by causing a minor and entirely safe degree of subclinical irritation

Warning: Before applying mask to the face, test a small amount on the skin of the arm for fifteen minutes to determine whether or not it's too irritating for you.

What you need:

(1) a small, deep bowl (ideal diameter: 6 inches)
(2) 1 60-gram tube of Lassar's Paste (a drugstore item made mostly of zinc oxide; use only *half* the tube.)
(3) 1 teaspoon alum (from your druggist)
(4) 3 teaspoons water

ZIZMOR'S RUBIFACTANT MASK

(5) ¼ cup rubifactant of your choice (mashed fresh strawberries or pineapple are two of my favorites)

(6) 1 teaspoon pectin (an optional gelling ingredient to make the mask a little stickier, available in foodstores)

Instructions: Combine ingredients in the bowl with the fingers. Apply to the face with the fingers, leaving clear areas around the eyes, nostrils, and mouth. Use it all; it won't keep. Allow to dry (usually five to ten minutes), and wash off with lukewarm water.

Special effects: A rubifactant mask is only slightly epiabrasive. Its effect is caused by your skin's reaction to the rubifactant substance. This kind of mask should not be used on a daily basis, as it may prove too irritating; like a dermatologist's mini-peel (which employs strong acids), rubifactant masks are meant for use before special occasions when you want to look your best. The slight subcutaneous swelling it causes is only temporary, but, while it lasts, it will plump up wrinkles and give the skin a smoother look. The plumping effect is mild and fleeting—albeit flattering—and will vanish in a few days.

CHAPTER 15

Grooming Implements and Appliances

Not very long ago Clairol, Inc. introduced a gizmo called the "face machine." I have a high regard for Clairol products, but the face machine, with its electrified whirling scrub-brush, is just the last word in commercial cosmetic nonsense. It may be electric, but I don't think it's a bit better than a regular old soapy washcloth—and it's considerably more expensive.

The machine has been selling well, of course, proving once again that gimmicks are good business even if they aren't always good sense. My feeling has always been that simple is best; I'm suspicious of needless automation and/or devices contrived to do very specialized jobs. And it's in this light that I'm going to evaluate popular grooming implements and appliances in the following categories:

    Hair Brushes
    Combs
    Cosmetic Scissors, Nippers, and Tweezers
    Files
    The Comedo Extractor
    Perma Tweez
    Electric Hair Rollers
    Curling Irons
    Blow Driers

Hair Brushes

There are more different types and styles of hair brushes than the human race can possibly use. But that doesn't stop people from constantly trying new ones—often in the misguided belief that only an expensive and highly specialized brush can perform satisfactorily. This is just baloney.

Probably the first question that comes to most minds concerns bristle type. Just what are "natural" bristles, and are they to be preferred over "synthetic" nylon bristles? "Natural" bristles come from wild boars, and brush manufacturers pick them up at auctions. Since wild boars seldom exist anywhere near civilized brush factories, natural bristles must all be imported—at considerable cost. Brush makers will tell you that natural bristles are superior because of their supposed "compatability" with human hair. All this means is that boar bristles are just another type of hair, albeit considerably tougher than our own. Bristles have cuticles (the protective miniature shingles that cover the outer surface of a hair) and imbrications (the openings between these cuticles), and some manufacturers claim that their uneven surface can better clean dust and dirt from human hair. It is also often implied by brush salespeople that the stiffness of natural bristles will somehow better stimulate the scalp and even distribute natural oils more efficiently.

Well, to expect a hair brush—natural or not—to clean dust and dirt from the hair is patently ridiculous. If your hair is dirty, don't brush it, wash it! As for stimulation of the scalp, this has no bearing at all on the health or appearance of the hair. Synthetic bristles do tend to be more flexible (therefore presumably less "stimulating") than natural varieties, but so what? A brush should have bristles strong enough to pass easily through the hair—and that's all. As for the distribution of natural scalp oils, this is a critical function of brushing, but there is no evidence to suggest that smooth, synthetic bristles distribute scalp oil any less efficiently than coarse, natural ones. Conclusion: there is no inherent advantage to natural bristles. As long as your brush is strong enough to go through your hair easily, any type of bristle will do.

How about the size and shape of your brush? This is another region filled with misleading advice. You can, of course, give yourself a case of temporary hair loss, or "traction alopecia," if you overuse a brush that is too heavy or too strong bristled for your hair. (You simply yank out hairs that aren't yet ready to naturally shed.) But don't fret too much about using the wrong type of brush; if it feels comfortable, then chances are it's perfectly suitable for your hair. And whether it's oval or squared or has a handle or not doesn't really matter. The one possible exception applies to women who brush their (usually long) hair with a final twist of the wrist; a round or half-round brush will wear better over the years.

There is nothing wrong with natural-bristle brushes except their price. They work just as well as the synthetics, and they usually have rather more attractive handles. But that doesn't make them worth the substantial extra cost. They must also be cared for more attentively. To clean them you must carefully comb caught hairs out from between the bristles, which must then be cleaned in tepid, soapy water. Special care must be taken to keep the wooden handle dry during both washing and rinsing of bristles lest it warp, crack, or mildew. And then the brush must be dried near an open window, but never in the sunshine or over a radiator—again for the sake of the handle. None of these precautions is necessary with typical synthetic-bristle brushes, since the handles are almost always made of plastic.

GROOMING IMPLEMENTS AND APPLIANCES

Further random observations on hair brushes: Does the color of the bristle make any difference? Only if you use a color rinse on your hair, in which case light bristles may become discolored. Does thin hair require special bristles? Yes; the thinner the hair, the softer the bristle should be. How often should you use a hair brush? Often enough to keep your hair attractively styled, but do beware of traction alopecia. Brushing a hundred strokes a day is a horrible idea; twenty-five is more than enough to efficiently distribute natural oils through the longest head of hair. What's the best way to brush? Sit down, lower your head, and brush forward first from the back of the scalp and then from the temples. When your oils are all distributed, put your head up and finish the brushing from the temples and the hairline back.

You can pay between $25 and $40 for a 100% pure boar-bristle brush made by firms like KENT OF LONDON or MASON PEARSON (also of London). I guess they make beautiful gifts. You can buy cheaper (because they're softer) natural-bristle brushes like the KINGSLEY 100% NATURAL BOAR BRISTLE (by Harry D. Koenig & Co.) and the SCALPMASTER 100% PURE BOAR BRISTLE (by Scalpmaster of France). These cost $4 to $5—better, but still expensive for a brush.

It's also possible to buy brushes made from a combination of nylon and boar bristle. The aforementioned Kent and Mason Pearson companies, for example, both carry combinations at prices well below those of their pure-bristle models. Yet, they're still expensive, and, from the standpoint of hair care, I can see no particular logic in combining bristle types. It's just a cost-cutting device.

Medically and economically speaking, a plastic-handled brush with nylon bristles is your all-around best bet. My favorites are the PRO STYLING BRUSH or the PRO FLAIR STYLE HAIRBRUSH, both by Vistron-Pro and each priced at well under two dollars. Each brush has a different bristle arrangement; the latter is mainly for short- or medium-length curly hair. I would give the same recommendation to any similar plastic and nylon brush.

Combs

Many people don't need brushes at all. They keep their hair neat and their scalp oils properly distributed simply by using a comb. But, alas, combs are like brushes in that many of them are ridiculously overpriced for no valid reason.

What makes a good comb? Teeth that are blunt, not too closely spaced, and strong enough not to break with normal combing. Bad combs have sharp teeth that can fracture the hair shafts and needlessly scratch the scalp. They have teeth so closely spaced that traction alopecia (the temporary hair loss described above) can result from normal daily grooming. And, since most good combs are cheap as well as strong, there's just no reason to get stuck with a brittle one.

My top recommendation goes to the ACE HARD RUBBER BARBER COMB (by Ace Comb Co.), which costs less than a dollar, is strong, and is ideally designed to slip easily through the hair. Ace also makes the long LADY ACE DRESSING COMB (all widely spaced teeth with no handle). It too gets my top recommendation. Combs cheaper than Ace are likely to break, and those that are more expensive literally offer nothing to justify the added cost.

Cosmetic Scissors, Nippers, and Tweezers

Speaking of added cost, it's possible to spend a shocking amount on highly specialized scissors and nippers. Is this necessary? Not at all.

First off, whether you use a pair of scissors or a barrel-spring nipper to trim your nails and cuticles is strictly up to you. Neither implement is superior. Both are sold in drug and department stores, sometimes for very fancy prices. I can't see spending $6.50 for nail nippers. So if you prefer a nipper—as I do—then ask the druggist or salesperson for the least expensive one. Luxury nippers don't cut nails any better than cheap ones.

As for scissors, I recommend the CUTICAL NAIL SCISSOR (by the La Cross division of A. R. Winarick, Inc.), because it combines nail and cuticle care in one implement. At about $5.50, this tool isn't cheap, but it's well engineered and correctly angled for a good, clean cut. And it has the virtue of being an all-in-one product that will satisfactorily perform nearly any task that requires cosmetic scissors.

I also recommend the KURLASH DELUXE TWISSORS (by Kurlash Co.), which are tweezers with scissors handles and cost less than $1.50. It's possible to spend almost four times this amount for a pair of tweezers, but it's pointless to do so. The "twissors" are not only good for regular tweezing, they also make putting on false eyelashes much easier and can be conveniently used on the eyebrows even when eyeglasses are worn.

Good traditional tweezers are made by Revlon and Maybelline and are sold at an even lower price than the Kurlash Twissors. You can usually find them with either straight or slanted ends. I prefer the slanted ones, but that's just a matter of personal preference and the way I hold my tweezers.

By the way, according to makeup artist Way Bandy (in his book *Designing Your Face*), the arch of the eyebrow should repeat the shape of the upper eyelid when you're looking straight into your makeup mirror.

Files

First of all, the purpose of nail files is not to cut or trim the nails. These implements are meant *only* to tidy up nails that have been freshly cut with scissors or nippers. Nail files are about as safe as any implement can be—unless they are overused. In that case, there is some minimal danger of a dirty file causing infection in tissue accidentally abraded by unnecessary filing.

There is no inherent difference between metal files and wooden emery boards. Nor is there much difference between files for the hands and files for the feet (the latter are simply bigger than fingernail files).

GROOMING IMPLEMENTS AND APPLIANCES

All wooden emery boards are equally effective. Among metal files, I recommend the LA CROSS FILE (by the La Cross division of A. R. Winarick, Inc.) because of its handy small size and sensible low price (well under a dollar).

The Comedo Extractor

Not too many people own one of these little tools. But if you have any acne—even if only occasionally—I'd recommend getting one. "Comedo" is the dermatological term for a pimple. The extractor, which looks at first glance like something from a dentist's office, is a slender stainless-steel implement with a point at one end and a tiny spoon with a hole in it at the other. It's what professional cosmetologists use, and it's a great improvement over squeezing pimples with the fingers.

To use the comedo extractor requires a little dexterity that anyone can easily develop. The pointed end is used to nick off the top of the pimple. This is called "deroofing." Then the spooned end is placed over the deroofed comedo and pressed in a slightly sidewise manner so as to squeeze out the trapped matter.

Opening a pimple this way definitely speeds healing. And using a comedo extractor makes successful opening and emptying relatively easy. Botching the job, as often happens with the fingers, forces irritating bacterial byproducts from within the pimple to go yet deeper into the surrounding tissue. This makes the irritation worse and the pimple bigger and redder.

Of course, the best way to fight acne flareups is to keep the skin clean and the pores unclogged. However, having some pimples is inevitable, and the comedo extractor, used properly, will definitely speed the healing process. Revlon makes a good extractor for about $2. If your favorite drug or department store doesn't have one, check the yellow pages for a surgical supply store.

Perma Tweez

This little appliance is an alternative to expensive professional electrolysis. It looks like a stubby fountain pen with a battery in the barrel and a little electrified tweezer at the tip. The Perma Tweez electrically shocks the follicle of each unwanted hair and in the process both removes the hair and destroys the follicle's ability to grow hair in the future.

Well, actually it doesn't destroy *every* follicle. The advertising leads you to believe that the product removes hair forever, but no form of electrolysis is 100% effective. Yet, even though some hairs are bound to grow back, the Perma Tweez will substantially reduce their number.

Perma Tweez is ideal for small areas (between the brows, above the lip, on the arms or breast) but not suitable for large areas with lots of hair, like legs or forearms. It does not puncture the skin, and it's entirely safe. However, it hurts—not excruciatingly, but enough to make it unpleasant.

Perma Tweez is sold through the mail for about $20 by a firm called General Medical Co., 1935 Armacost Ave., West Los Angeles, California 90025. It's regularly advertised in the back pages of beauty and fashion magazines, and I give it a high recommendation.

Electric Hair Rollers

Electric rollers are a fairly speedy way to set hair in temporary curls. Their combination of heat and moisture sets hair as well as if you spent an entire night in rollers or pincurls.

There's no electricity in the individual rollers. They come together in a carrier box that wets and heats them, after which they are individually rolled into the hair. How well do they work? Quite well. Do they work equally well for everybody? No. They work best for people who have a good haircut plus a little practice in roller placement. How long will the set last? Until the next shampoo (or rainstorm, if you get caught in it). How long should electric rollers be left in the hair? Until the hair is completely cooled. Can electric rollers hurt your hair? No, they're not hot enough. Who makes recommended electric roller sets? Clairol and General Electric.

Curling Irons

Curling irons, unlike electric rollers, definitely can hurt your hair. The damage doesn't happen all at once, but if you use one every day, slowly you'll ruin the cuticle layer of your hair. That's because the excessive heat generated by a curling iron progressively dehydrates the cuticle and leads to permanently opened imbrications. When that happens, the hairs won't slide against one another easily and will appear dull and lusterless. Eventually, the cuticles at the ends can rub off altogether, causing unattractive and unmanageable split ends.

Using a curling iron occasionally before a dressy event won't hurt you at all. The danger lies in the temptation to use one every day to add curls and flips. It's easy to succumb, since today's curling irons are light and easy to use, won't stick to the hair, and impart a good curl instantaneously. Some even come with special misting attachments, which aren't necessary but do make the curls a bit stronger.

If you buy a curling iron, be sure to get one that's approved by Underwriters' Laboratories. This at least assures you that the appliance is safely wired. Of the many irons on the market, I recommend the LADY SCHICK QUICK CURLS, Clairol's CRAZY CURL, and the OSTER MIST SET. But this is a recommendation for limited and occasional use *only*.

Blow Driers

People love blow driers, even though they're worse for the hair than curling irons. Everything a curling iron can do to the hair cuticles, a blow drier can do, too—except more so. Although it may seem wonderfully convenient to dry, style,

GROOMING IMPLEMENTS AND APPLIANCES

and add a static-electric fullness to the hair in one easy step, an unfortunate price must eventually be paid.

Since blow-drier damage is a gradual and cumulative affair, people tend to ignore it until it's too late. However, the day will dawn when you can no longer overlook your fried cuticles and your hair will look like a wretched thatch. This is the inevitable fate of hair submitted daily to the excessive heat of a blow drier.

What can you do to avoid it? First, use a blower for special occasions only and don't depend on it for your daily style. Next, if you must get a drier, get one with less than 1000 watts of power. (The wattage is clearly printed on the appliance itself.) If you insist on using your blower every time you shampoo, a lower-watted model will at least cause less damage to the hair shafts. Finally, you can protect your cuticles to a certain degree by coating them with protein. A regular conditioner is, however, not quite enough. You can insulate your cuticles better from the damaging heat of the blower with a special heat-activated, blow-drier conditioner such as THE HEAT SOLUTION (by Pantene), KINDNESS or ZAP (both by Clairol), or BLOW-CARE (by Cosmetco). Don't expect these products to protect the hair completely; they just mitigate the damage somewhat.

I'm hard pressed to recommend appliances of which I don't really approve. General Electric, Clairol, Remington, Schick, Sunbeam, and any number of other manufacturers make blowers that are excellent from a mechanical standpoint, even though regular use of any one of them is bad for your hair. Medically speaking, you should let your hair dry naturally.

Index

Abbot Labs, 124
Ace Hard Rubber Barber Comb, 174
Acetone, 110
Acidity, 11–12
Acnaveen, 146
Acne, 69, 142–148; causes of, 142–143; cold cream and, 23, 78, 79; epiabrading, 26; formation of pimples, 143–144; makeup, 94, 96; medicines for, 144–148; squeezing pimples, 148
Acne-Aid Detergent Soap, 146
Acne Cream, 144
Acqua di Selva, 45
Adorn Self-Styling Hair Spray, 136
Advertising claims, 1, 5–6, 18
A-Fil Cream, 162
Afro-Sheen, 129
Aftate Antifungal, 152
Aftershave lotions, 35–37, 41, 42
Aftersun moisturizers, 165–166
Agree Creme Rinse & Conditioner, 127
Aim, 86–87
Aime Lipbleach, 141
Alberto Culver: Alberto Balsam Shampoo, 121; Alberto VO 5, see Alberto VO 5; Consort Hair Spray for Men, 136; Get Set Setting Lotion, 132
Alberto VO 5: Conditioning Hairdressing, 131; Gentle as Rain Water Shampoo, 121; Hairspray, 136; Miral Plus Hairspray for Improved Holding, 135; Non-Aerosol Hairspray, 135; Whipped Creme Rinse & Conditioner, 127
Alkalinity, 11–12, 119
Allantoin, 71, 73, 74, 121
Allergic reaction: allergenic ingredients, 7; to artificial nails, 111; to benzocaine, 166, 167; industry testing and, 2–3; to makeup, 92, 93; to nail polish, 102–103; to perfumes and colognes, 42, 43, 44; to scented soap, 21; sensitization and, 1–2, 6
All-purpose compress, 9
Almay: Cheq Roll-On Antiperspirant Deodorant, 62; Color 'N Gleam, 102; Color Rich Eye Shadow, 103; Cover Up Stick, 98; Creme Nail Enamel, 109; Creme Tint Lipsticks, 101; Deep Mist Cleansing Lotion, 80; Deep Mist Moisture Lotion, 70; Eyebrow Pencil With Built-In

Almay (cont'd)
Sharpener, 106; face powders by, 98–99; Fineline Eye Pencil, 106; Hair Mist, 135; Hypoallergenic Cold Cream, 79; Protective Base Coat, 113; Semi-Filter Sun Lotion, Full-Filter Sun Lotion, and Deep Tanning Oil, 161; shampoos by, 122; Sketchstix Creme Shadow Pencil, 106; Sun Bloc Gel, Deep Tanning Cream, and Semi-Filter Sun Creme, 162; Toning Lotion for Oily Skin, 82; Under Eye Cover Creme, 98; Whip Creme Blush, 100
Alo: After Tan, 166; Fashion Tan Suntan Moisturizer, 163; Sun Block Lotion, 163; Super Rich Tan, 163
Aloe, 163–164
Aloe Creme Labs. See Alo
Aloise Nail Polish, 109
Alpha Keri: Bath Oil, 18, 24; Soap, 18
Aluminum chlorohydrate, 58, 60
Aluminum sulphate, 35
American Safety Razor Co., 31
Andrea Fresh-Ups, 106
Androgen, 142–143
Angle Synton, 89
Antibiotics, for acne, 147–148
Anti-gray products, 136–137
Anti-perspirants: foot, 150, 151; underarm, 58–63
Apollo Sun for a Safe, Dark Tan, 162
Après Le Soleil, 166
Aquacre, 68, 110, 165; HP, 68
Aquamarine Moisture Cream, 70
Aquaphore, 100, 101
Aqua Velva: Ice Blue or Redwood, 36; Silicone Lather Shave, 34
Aramis: after shave lotion, 37; colognes by, 45–46; moisturizers by, 74; 900, see also Aramis 900; shampoos by, 122
Aramis 900: Absolute Comfort Shave Foam, 34; Concentrated Anti-perspirant Spray
Arm & Arm With Baking Soda Deodorant, 59
Arm & Hammer Baking Soda Deodorant with Cornstarch, 59
Arpege: Eau liquid cologne, 54; Moisturizing Body Lotion, 76
Arrid: Cream Deodorant, 62; Extra Antiperspirant Pump Spray, 61; Extra Dry Antiperspirant Spray, 61; Extra Dry Antiperspirant

Arrid (cont'd)
Spray-Light Powder, 62; Extra Dry Roll-On Antiperspirant Deodorant, 62; XX Extra Extra Dry New Formula Antiperspirant Spray, 61
Artificial nails, 111
Artistry II Beauty Scrub Cleansing Treatment, 23
Artra Skin Tone Cream, 81
Astringents, 81–82
Athlete's foot, 151–152
Aveeno Colloidal Oatmeal, 24–25
Aviance: Body Lotion, 76; Cologne, 56; Perfume, 50
Avocado oil, 72
Avon: bath oil and bead products by, 25; Clear Skin Soap, 15; Rich Moisture Bath Bar, 18
Aziza: mascara by, 105; Natural Lustre Lip Gloss, 102

Baby Soft Body Lotion, 76
Bacitracin, 154
Bad breath, 84, 86, 87–88
Bain de Soleil Suntan Lotion, 162; Super Filter, 162
Baldness, 116–117
Balsam, 121
Ban: Basic Non-Aerosol Antiperspirant Spray, 61; Quick Dry Roll-On Antiperspirant Deodorant, 62; Roll-On Antiperspirant Deodorant, 62; Ultra Ban Antiperspirant Lotion, 62; Ultra Ban 5000, 61
Bandy, Way, 93, 175
Barbasol: Brushless Shave Cream, 33; Concentrated Lather Shaving Cream, 34
Bare-Face, 145
Barth's Sea Gel, 87
Basis Soap, 18
Bath brushes, 27
Batherapy, 25
Bathing, 11–29
Bath oils, 23–26
Bath salts, 24
Bathwater additives, 23–26
Beauty grains, 23
Beecham Products. See Brylcreem
Beeswax, 71, 75, 98
Beiersdorf, Inc., 68
Bellodgia: Parfum de toilette, 52; Perfume, 49
Benadryl, 167
Benoxyl-5 Lotion and Benoxyl-10 Lotion, 145
5-Benzagel and 10-Benzagel, 144
Benzethonium chloride, 64

179

INDEX

Benzocaine, 34, 71, 153, 166–167
Benzoyl peroxide, 144, 145, 146
Berloque dermatitis, 42, 43
Betadine Douche, 64
BHA, 7
BHT, 7
Bic Shaver, 31
Bill Blass, 45
Bio Products, 147
Bleaches: facial hair, 141; hair, 137–138; skin (bleaching creams), 80–81
Blondit, 141
Blow Care, 178
Blow driers, 177–178
Blue Carnation: Eau de toilette, 56; Perfume, 50
Blushers, 99–100
Body lotions, creams, and ointments, 66–67, 75–76
Bonne Belle: Colorado Colors Spring Eyeshadows, 103; Honest Makeup, 96; Medicated Masque, 169; True Blush, 100
Boric acid, 27, 64
Brace, 91
Braggi: after shave lotion, 37; cologne, 46
Bravura, 37
Breck: Beautiful Hair Breck Creme Rinse, 127; Breck Basic: Conditioner With Protein, 128; Breck Beautiful Clean Rinse, 127; Hair Color, 139; Miss Breck: Lasting Hold Non-Aerosol Hair Spray, 134; Set Setting Lotion, 133
Bristol Myers Co. *See* Score; Vitalis
British Sterling: after shave lotion, 37; cologne, 47
Brushes: bath, 27; hair, 172–174
Brut 33: cologne, 45; Creme Shave, 34; Hair Control Spray, 136; Pre-Electric Shave, 30
Brylcreem, 131; Blue Brylcreem for Grey Hair, 131; green-formula, 132; Soft Hair, 136
Buf, 147
Buf Puf, 23, 26, 153, 168

Cabochard: Eau de toilette, 54; Perfume, 48
Caesar, 47
Caladryl Lotion, 167
Calandre by Paco Rabanne, 48
Calcium pantothenate, 121
Caleche: Eau de toilette, 52; Perfume, 48
Calgon: Bath Oil Beads, 24; Bouquet Bath, 24
Calluses, 153
Camay, 15
Canoe, 46
Cantharone, 158
Capricci: Eau de toilette, 55; Perfume, 49
Capucci "Pour Home," 45
Caress, 17, 19
Carmol, 68

Caron Parfums: colognes by, 45, 46, 52, 53; perfumes by, 48, 49
Carson Product Co., 35
Carter-Wallace, 38
Caryl Richards: Balsam Plus Protein Instant Hair Conditioner, 127; Just Wonderful Hairspray, 135
Castile soaps, 15
Castor oil, 17, 72
Celebrity, 106
Ceresin, 79
Cerissa: Concentrated Cologne, 52; Perfume, 47
Cetyl alcohol, 71, 72, 74
Chamade: Cologne, 53; Perfume, 48
Chanel: after shave lotion by, 37; lip glosses by, 102; masks by, 170; for Men, 46; moisturizers by, 74; nail polishes by, 109
Chanel No. 5: Body Lotion, 76; Eau de toilette, 54; Perfume, 50
Chanel No. 19: Body Lotion, 76; Eau de toilette, 54; Perfume, 50
Chanel No. 22: Eau de cologne, 55; Perfume, 50
Chant D'Aromes: Cologne, 53; Perfume, 49
Chantilly: Eau de toilette, 55; Perfume, 50
Chapstick, 100, 101; Face Quencher, 96
Charles of the Ritz, 6; masks by, 170; nail polishes by, 109; Revenescence Lipstick, 101; Revenescence Powderglow, 99; Wholesome Makeup All-Day Face Tint, 97
Charles Revson: Basic Makeup Oil-Blotting Formula, 95; C. H. Revson Extraordinary Face Makeup, 97; colognes by, 46, 51, 52; perfumes by, 47
Charlie: Cologne, 55; Extra Extra Shine Lipstick, 101; Perfume, 51
Chaz, 46
Checkmate Deodorant Antiperspirant, 62
Cheek-Glo Rouge, 100
Cheek glosses and blushers, 99–100
Chesebrough-Pond's, Inc. *See* Vaseline
Chloe: Eau de Toilette, 51; Perfume, 47
Christian Dior: colognes by, 46, 52, 54; Eau Sauvage. *See* Eau Sauvage; Lipstick, 101; perfumes by, 48
Chromatics, 45
Ciara, 47
Ciara 100, 51
Cie: Lavish Cologne, 56; Perfume, 50
Cinoxate, 163
Citric acid, 121, 132
Clairol: Balsam Color, 139; blow driers by, 178; Born Blond Lightener, 137; Clairoxide Liq-

Clairol *(cont'd)*
uid Developer, 137; Conditioning Beauty Pack Treatment, 128; Crazy Curl, 177; electric roller sets by, 177; Final Net, 132, 134; Hair So New Creme Rinse, 128; Happiness, 139; Herbal Essence, 121; Herbal Essence Creme Rinse, 127; Instant Condition Treatment, 127; Kindness Instant Protein Hair Conditioner, 128, 178; Lemon Go Lightly, 138; Long & Silky Conditioning Lotion for Long Hair, 127; Loving Care Color Foam, 139; Loving Care Hair Color Lotion, 139; Miss Clairol Hair Color Bath Creme Formula, 139; Nice 'N Easy, 139; Picture Perfect Color Rinse, 140; Power Pal Conditioning Styling Mist for Blow Drying, 128; Short & Sassy, 121; Short & Sassy Conditioning Lotion, 127; Summer Blond, 138; Sunshine Harvest Shampoo, 122; Zap, 178
Clarity Beauty Beads, 23
Cleansers, cream, 13, 78–80
Clearasil: Acne Pimples Cream Medication, 145, 146; Antibacterial Acne Lotion, 144; Medicated Cleanser, 147
Clinique: Allergy Tested Base Coat and Allergy Tested Top Glaze, 113; Antiperspirant Deodorant Roll-on, 62; Basic Eye Emphasizer, 105; cheek blushers by, 100; Concealing Stick, 98; Continuous Coverage, 97; Different Lipstick, 102; Extremely Gentle Cleansing Cream, 80; Extremely Smoothing Body Lotion, 76; face powders by, 99; Herb Shampoo, 123; lip glosses by, 102; mascaras by, 105; masks by, 170; Men's Face Soap, 15; moisturizers by, 74; nail polishes by, 109; Re-Moisturizing Lipstick, 102; shampoos by, 121; Soap Extra Strength, 15; Soap Mild, 19; Softly Sheer, 99; Special Hand and Body Lotion, 76; Transparent Buffer, 99
Close-Up, 86–87
Coast, 20
Cocoa butter, 72
Coconut oil, 17, 19, 20, 34
Cold creams, 22–23, 78–80
Colgate: Cup Soap for Shaving, 33; Instant Shave, 34; Tooth Paste, 87; Tooth Powder, 87
Colognes, 36, 37, 41–47; for men, 45–47; for women, 51–56
Coloring agents, 7
Comb Easy Hair Conditioner Lotion, 129
Combs, 174–175
Comedo extractors, 148, 176
Compress, all-purpose, 9
Concealers, 97–98

180

INDEX

Conditioners, hair, 124–129, 178
Confident, 91
Contemporary Fragrance Group. *See* Cie
Conti Castile Soap, 15
Coombe, Inc., 137
Cooper Labs, 146
Coppertone: Suntan Lotion, Suntan Oil, and Tanning Butter, 163; Super Shade Sunblocking Lotion, 162, 163; Tan Care, 166
Corega, 90
Corn-O-Cide Medicated Foot Bath, 153
Cosmetico, 178
Coty: Away Mask, 169; Glowing Finish All In One Makeup, 96; Glowing Finish Cremepowder Blush, 100; Nature's Blush, 100; Nuance. *See* Nuance; Silksticks, 101
Courtesy Bubbling Bath Oil, 25
Cover Girl: All Day Oil Control Makeup, 95; Clean Makeup, 96; Lip Softeners, 101; Long 'N Lush Mascara, 105; Moisture Wear Liquid Moisture Makeup, 96; "Nail Slicks," 109; One Stroke Eye Color, 103; Sheer Makeup, 95; Shine Maker, 102
Creams, 66–67, 75–81; *See also* Moisturizers
Creme rinses, 126
Crepe de Chine: Eau de toilette concentrate, 55; Soap, 21
Crest, 86–87
Curling irons, 177
Cushion Grip, 91
Cutex Oily Nail Polish Remover, 110
Cutical Nail Scissor, 175
Cuticle removers, 113
Cuticle treatments, 111–112

Daisy Twin Blade Shaver, 31
Dana Perfumes: cologne by, 46, 56; perfume by, 50
Dandruff: hair dressings, 131–132; shampoos, 123–124, 129
Demure Deodorant Douche Concentrate, 64
Dental floss, 83–85
Denture adhesives, 90–91
Denture cleaners, 89–90
Deodorants: foot, 149–150; soaps, 20–21; underarm, 58–60
DEP: Balsam DEP Super Hair Styling Gel, 133; Balsam Mist Protein Hair Conditioner, 127; Dry Styling Control, 130; For Men Dry Styling Hair Control, 136
Depilatories, 37–38
Dermassage Medicated Skin Lotion, 71
"Dermatologist tested" products, 3
Dermik Labs: acne preparations by, 144, 145, 146; Color Blender, 95

Desenex, 152; soap, 28
Designing Your Face (Bandy), 93, 175
Desquam-X 5 Gel and Desquam-X 10 Gel, 144
Detect Plaque Disclosing Tablets, 85
DHS Dermatological Hair and Scalp Shampoo, 123
Diagonal: Eau de toilette, 54; Perfume, 49
Dial: Soap, 20; Very Dry Roll-On Antiperspirant, 62; With Very Dry Antiperspirant, 61
Dihydroxy acetone, 164
Dimethyl amino benzoate, 163
Diorella: Eau de toilette, 52; Perfume, 48
Diorissimo: Eau de cologne, 54; Perfume, 48
Dippity-Do Setting Gel, 133
Disclosing tablets, 85
Dismiss Disposable Douche, 65
Dr. Lyon's Tooth Powder, 87
Dr. Scholl's: Bromidrosis Foot Powder, 151; Chlorophyll Foot Deodorant Powder, 151; Deodorant Refresher Spray, 150; Dry Antiperspirant Foot Spray, 151; Foot Powder, 150; Foot Powder Spray, 152; Leg Hair Remover, 38; Solvex Athlete's Foot Powder, 153; Solvex Athlete's Foot Spray, Spray Powder, and Pump Spray, 153
Dolomite, 87
Dorothy Gray: Basic Formula for Sensitive Skin, 70–71; Basic Formula Sensitive Skin Pure Cleanser, 79; Cellogen Moisturizing Hormone Cream, 77; Masque Frappé, 170; Moisturizing Hand Cream, 75; Moisturizing Salon Cold Cream, 79; Satura Moisture Cream with Vitamin A, 72; 2 Minute Magic Lotion, 80; Wax, 38
Douches, 63–65
Dove, 18
Dri-foot Deodorant Spray and Antiperspirant, 151
Drift, 47
Drücken brush, 27
Dry Look, The, 136; Liquid Hair Control, 131; Pump Spray, 135
DuBarry Cleansing Grains, 23
Duofilm, 158
Dyes, hair, 138–140
Dyshydrosis, 151

Earth Born pH Balanced Creme Rinse & Conditioner, 127
Easo: Denture Adhesive Powder, 90; Denture Cushions, 91
Eau de Calandre, 52
Eau Sauvage: aftershave, 37; cologne, 46; Spray Deodorant, 62
Eclipse Sunscreen Lotion, 162
Eczema, 27
Edema, 2
Edge Lathering Gel, 34

Efferdent, 90
Elder, Paul B., Co., 161
Electric hair rollers, 177
Electric razors, 29, 39–40
Elizabeth Arden, 93; moisturizers by, 74; Very Special Base Coat, 113
Email Diamant, 87
Emulsifiers, 7, 24, 95
End papers, 133–134
English Leather: after shave lotion, 37; cologne, 47; Powder Foam Shave Cream, 34
Epiabrasion, 26–27, 168
Epilators, 37, 38
Equipage, 45
Esotérica: bleaching cream, 81; Soap, 18
Estée Lauder: moisturizers by, 74; nail polishes by, 109; Re-Nutriv Rich Rich Lipstick, 101; Soap, 21
Estrogen, 77, 80
Ethanolamine, 15, 17
Etherea: Active Mud Masque, 170; Basic Makeup for Normal/Dry Skin, 97; cheek blushers by, 100; Complete Cleansing Lotion, 80; Fresh Skin, 169; lip glosses by, 102; mascaras by, 105; Moisturizing Eye Shadow Dual Plan, 104; nail polishes by, 109; Oil Control Cleansing Lotion, 80; Oil-Control Cleansing Soap, 19; Shining Lipstick, 102; Special Formula Lipstick, 102; Transparent Color Glaze, 97; Translucent Creme Makeup for Normal/Dry Skin, 97; Wrinkle Gelstick, 98
Eucerin, 68
Eye colors, 102–104
Eyelash adhesives, 106
Eye liners, 105
Eye pencils, 106
Eyeshadows, 102–104

Fabergé: All Purpose Aqua Net Professional Hair Spray, 136; Babe Country Cheek Colors, 100; Babe Country Face Colors, 96; Babe Country Lip Colors, 101; Babe Eye Shadow, 103; Brut 33. *See* Brut 33; Caryl Richards. *See* Caryl Richards; Fabergé Lipstick, 101; Fabergé Organics Pure Wheat Germ Oil & Honey Conditioner, 127; Fabergé Organics Pure Wheat Germ Oil & Honey Shampoo, 121; Flatterlash Mascara, 105; Great Skin with NMC—12 Dry Care Moisturizer, 71; Liquid Nail Dry, 113; Nail Glaze, 109; Nail Glaze Remover, 110; Peach A La Mode Milk Protein Shampoo With Nucleic Acid, 112
Face blotters, 106
Face powders, 94, 98–99
Facial hair bleaches, 141

181

INDEX

Facial masks, 168–171
Fanci-Full Rinse, 140
Fantasia Industries Corp., 130
Farouche: Eau de toilette, 55; Perfume, 48
Fasteeth Denture Adhesive Powder, 90
Feet, 149–154
Feminine hygiene preparations, 63
Feminique: Deodorant Liquid Concentrate, 64; Disposable Douche, 65
Femme: Cologne regular, 54; Perfume, 49
Fingercots, 112
Five Day: Antiperspirant Deodorant Pads, 60; Non-Aerosol Antiperspirant, 61; Roll-On Antiperspirant, 62
Fixodent, 91
Flame Glo, 102
Fleurs de Rocaille: Parfum de toilette, 52; Perfume, 49
Flex: Balsam & Protein Instant Hair Conditioner, 127; Balsam and Protein Shampoo, 121; Hair Net, 135; Non-Aerosol Hair Net, 132, 134; Setting Lotion, 133
Flicker, 31
Flori Roberts: Checkmate Deodorant Antiperspirant, 62; Liquid Glo, 100; Melana Soufflé, 95; Melanin Face Powder, 99; Melanin Makeup Base, 95
Flospik, 84–85
Floss Mate Dental Floss Handle, 84
Flowery Professional Nail White Pencil, 114
Fluorocarbon propellants, 134
Folliculitis, 35
Foreplay Suntan Lotion and Suntan Oil, 164
Formula 405: Bath Oil, 25; Deep Action Moisturizer, 71; Soap, 18
Fortifiers, nail, 112–113
Fostex, 147; CM, 146
Fostril Drying Lotion for Acne, 146
Foundation makeups, 94–97
Fragrance soaps, 21–22
Frances Denney, 96
Fresh: Cream Antiperspirant Deodorant, 62; Non-Stinging Antiperspirant Deodorant, 61; Stick Antiperspirant Deodorant, 62
Fuller Complexion Brush, 26
Fungal infections, 13, 28, 108, 151–153

Gelatin, 107, 121, 129
General Electric: blow driers by, 178; electric roller sets by, 177
Geoffrey Beene, 45
Gillette: Adorn Self-Styling Hair Spray, 136; Blue Blades, 32; Brushless Shave Cream, 33; Dippity-Do Setting Gel, 133; Disposable Twin Blade Razor,

Gillette (cont'd)
31; Earth Born pH Balanced Creme Rinse & Conditioner, 127; Foamy, 34; Foot Guard, Foot Deodorant and Dry Spray Powder, 151; Foot Guard Antifungal Foot Deodorant Medicated Foot Care, 153; Heads Up Hair Groom, 131; Lather Shave Cream, 33; Maxi Hold Super Holding Hair Spray, 135; Platinum Plus Blades, 31; Platinum Plus Injector Blades, 31–32; Superadjustable, 30; Super Blue Blades, 32; Super Stainless Blades, 32; Tame Creme Rinse & Conditioner, 127; Techmatic, 31; The Dry Look. *See* Dry Look, The; The Hot One, 34; Toni, 141; Trac II Blades, 31, 32; Trac II Shave Cream, 34; Twinjector Blades, 32
Ginseng: Cologne Concentrate Spray, 55; Perfume, 51
Ginseng for Men: Jovan, Inc., 46; MEM Co., Inc., 47
Givenchy: Gentleman, 45; Gentleman Deodorant Anti-Perspirant Spray, 62
Givenchy III: Eau de toilette, 52; Perfume, 48
Gleem, 87
Glosses: cheek, 99–100; lip, 100, 102
Glycerine, 7, 17, 23, 34, 35, 36, 68, 71, 75
Glycerine soaps, 18–19
Glycerol stearates, 72, 74
Goodman, H., & Son, Inc., 134
Grecian Formula 16, 137
Grey Flannel, 45
Groom & Clean Greaseless Hair Control, 131
Grooming implements and appliances, 172–178
Guerlain: colognes by, 53; perfumes by, 48, 49, 50

Hair brushes, 172–174
Hair care and coloring products, 119–141
Hair driers, 177–178
Hair removal, 37–38
Hair rollers, electric, 177
Hair structure and growth, 115–118
Halston: colognes by, 45; Lipstick, 101; Milk Bath Powder, 25; Soap, 21
Hand lotion, 66–67, 75
Hard As Nails With Nylon, 109
Head & Shoulders Shampoo, 124
Helena Rubinstein: Bio-Clear, 169; Brush-On-Peel-Off Mask, 169; Cream Care and Frost Care Lipsticks, 101; Deep Cleanser, 79; Fresh Cover Blushing Cream, 100; Fresh Cover Liquid Makeup, 95; Gloss Care, 102; Long Lash Mascara, 105; Min-

Helena Rubinstein (cont'd)
ute Liquid Liner, 105; Nudit. *See* Nudit; "Pasteurized" Face Cream Special, 77; Strong and Glossy, 113; Strong & Icy, 109
Helene Curtis: Everynight Balsam & Protein Shampoo, 121; Everynight Herb Shampoo, 122; Suave: Balsam & Protein Instant Hair Conditioner, 128
Henna, 140
Herbal, 45
Herbert Labs, 124, 162
Hoffritz Angle Razor, 30
Home permanents, 140–141
Honey, 23
Hopkins Company, 140
Houbigant: colognes by, 46, 47, 55; Hand and Body Moisturizer, 71; perfume by, 50
House of Fragrance, Inc., 55
Humectants, 86, 95
Humidifiers, 67
Hydrogenated vegetable oil, 70, 73, 75
Hydrogen peroxide, 137
Hydrolized animal protein, 74, 121, 126, 129, 132
Hydroquinone, 80–81
Hypoallergenic products, 1–3, 6

Infini: Parfum de toilette, 52; Perfume, 48
Ingrown toenails, 154
Inner Rinse Liquid Douche Concentrate, 64
Integra face powders, 99
Int'l Perfumes Ltd., 46
Iocon Shampoo Tar Gel Concentrate for Dandruff Control, 124
Ionax: Scrub, 147; Shampoo for Oily Hair & Scalp, 121; Foam, 147
Ionil: Nonionic/Cationic Therapeutic Dandruff Shampoo, 124; T Nonionic/Cationic Therapeutic Dandruff Shampoo, 124; Rinse Conditioner, 129
Irish Spring, 20–21
Isopropyl myristate, 30
Isopropyl palmitate, 70, 71
Ivory, 14, 15

Jacqueline Cochran, Inc., 45
Jade East, 47
Jean Marie Forina, 46
Jean Naté: Antiperspirant Spray, 61; For Men After Shave, 37; Friction pour le bain, 56; Roll-On Antiperspirant, 62
Jean Patou: cologne by, 51; perfume by, 47
Jergen: Bubbling Bath Beads, 25; "Gee Your Hair Smells Terrific" Shampoo, 122; Pre Heat Protective Conditioner, 128; Soap, 18
Jergen's Lotion, 71; Direct Aid Hand Lotion, 75; for Extra Dry Skin Keri Cream, 71; Hand Lotion, 75

INDEX

Jewel By Lady Schick, 39
Jicky: Perfume, 50; Toilet Water, 53
Johnson & Johnson: Baby Soap, 17; Deodorant Foot Powder, 149; Detect Plaque Disclosing Tablets, 85; See also Johnson's
Johnson's: Baby Cream, 76; Baby Lotion, 76; Baby Oil, 76; Odor Eaters, 150
Jolen Creme Bleach, 141
Jontue: Body Silk, 76; Cologne, 56; Perfume, 51
Jovan, Inc.: colognes by, 46, 55; perfumes by, 51
Joy: Eau de Joy, 51; Perfume, 47

Kanon: after shave lotion, 37; Cologne, 46; Man's Antiperspirant Spray Talc, 62; Rich Shave Foam, 34
Kent of London, 174
Kingsley 100% Natural Boar Bristle, 174
Kip First Aid Spray and Kip Sunburn Lotion, 167
Klaron Acne Lotion, 146
Kleenite, 90
Koenig, Harry D., & Co., 174
Komed Acne Lotion and Mild Komed Acne Lotion, 145
Kurlash Deluxe Twissors, 175

L T Laboratories, 137
La Cross: Cutical Nail Scissor, 175; File, 176
Lactona: denture adhesive, 90; Natural, 89; toothbrush, 89
Lady Ace Dressing Comb, 174–175
L'Air Du Temps: Eau de toilette, 55; Perfume, 49
Lanacaine Medicated Dry Skin Lotion, 71
Lancôme: mascaras by, 105; masks by, 170
Lanolin, 18, 19–20, 34, 35, 36, 68, 70–73, 75, 98, 110
Lanvin-Charles of the Ritz: Après Le Soleil, 166; Bain de Soleil. See Bain de Soleil; colognes by, 45, 54, 56; perfumes by, 50
Lanvin Modern Bath Salts, 25
Lauderdale Cosmetics, 164
Lava, 27
Lecithin, 80
Le De: Eau de toilette, 54; Perfume, 48
Lederle Labs, 124
Le Muguet de Bonheur: Parfum de toilette, 53; Perfume, 49
Lenel for Men, 46
Les Pois de Senteur: Parfum de toilette, 53; Perfume, 49
Lever Brothers Company, 17
Lewer Drug Products of New York City, 35
L'Heure Bleue: Cologne, 53; Perfume, 49
Lifebuoy, 14

Lilac Vegetal, 36
L'Interdit: Eau de toilette, 54; Perfume, 48
Lipsticks, 100–102
Listerex: Cleansing Gel, 147; Liquid, 147
Listerine, 86–87, 88
Loofah, 26–27
Loofah Mitt, 27
Loofah Natural Bath Sponge, 27
Loofah Strap, 27
L'Oreal: Creme Lip Accents, 101; Creme Nail Accents, 109; Excellence Extra Rich Hair Color, 139; Extra Body Perm, 141; Hold Straight, 133; Miracle Accents Miracle Base, 113; Naturally Free Setting Lotion, 132; Preference, 139; Satine Setting Lotion, 132; Shampoo, 121; Silk and Silver Color Lotion, 139; Suffrage Hair Spray, 135; Young Blond, 138
Loroxide Acne Lotion, 144
Love: Lovesticks, 101; Oil Free Gel Makeup, 95
Love's Fresh Lemon Fluffy Moisturizer, 70
Lowila, 27
Lubriderm, 70
Lush Lips, 102

Macho, 45
MacLeans, 86–87
Madame Jovan: Cologne Concentrate Spray, 55; Perfume, 51
Madame Rochas: Cologne regular, 54; Perfume, 49
Madrid Ltd., 130
Magic: Aftershave Skin Conditioner, 36; Cooling Soothing After Shave Cream, 36; Shaving Powder, 35
Maja: Perfume, 48; Soap, 21
Majestic Drug Co., 137
Makeup, 92–106
Mani Magic Cuticle Remover, 113
Mascaras, 104–105
Masks, 168–171
Mason Pearson, 174
Massage-Brush, 27
Massengill: Disposable Douche, 65; Douche Powder, 64; Liquid Douche, 64
Max Factor: Active Moisturizer, 70; Blue Mask, 169; Brush Tip Mascara, Maxi-Lash Mascara, Lash Full Mascara, 104; Creme-Puff Makeup, 96; Creme Shine Lip Color, 102; Erace, 98; Fine Line Automatic Eye Pencil, 106; Gentle Foam Cleanser, 79; Hi-Fi Eye Shadow Stick, 104; Hi-Fi Fluid Eye-Liner, 105; Hi-Fi Fluid Makeup, 96; Lash Maker Automatic Comb on Mascara, 104; Linemakers Stay On Liner, 105; Mascara Wand, 105; Maxi-Moist Lipstick, 101; Moisture Essence, 72; Moistur-

Max Factor (cont'd)
izing Liquid Cleanser, 80; Nail Polish Remover, 110; Pan Cake Makeup, 95–96; Pan Stick Makeup, 96, 98; Secret Key, 82; Self-Defense Moisturizer, 72; Super Clean Cleanser, 80; Super Clear Makeup with Lecithin, 96; Super Lash Maker Comb On, Brush On, Roll On Mascara, 104; Tried and True, 139; Ultra Lucent Oil-Free Pure Moisture Fluid Makeup, 95; Ultralucent Whipped Creme Blush, 100; Ultralucent Whipped Creme Lipstick, 101; Ultralucent Whipped Creme Nail Enamel, and Maxi-Wear Nail Guard, 109; Ultra Lucent Whipped Creme Pressed Powder, 99; Waterproof Eye Shadow, Creme-On Eye Shadow, Whipped Creme Enriched Eye Shadow, Maxi-Rich Shadow, 103; Yogurt Moisture Concentrate, 73
Maybelline, 6; Automatic Cream-On Shadow, Ultra Frost, Ultra Velvet, Pearly Ultra Frost, 103; Automatic Super Shiny Lip Color, 102; Brown Pencil, 106; Fresh & Lovely Moisture Whip, 96; Fresh & Lovely Oil Makeup, 95; Linear Pencil, 106; Lip Color, 101; Look Natural Comb-On Mascara, 104; Nail Color, 109; tweezers by, 175
Mazon Medicated Soap, 18
MEM Co., Inc., 47
Mennen: Afta After Shave Skin Conditioner, 36; Antiperspirant Spray Deodorant, 61; Baby Magic Lotion, 76; Brake Antiperspirant Roll-On, 62; Brushless Shave, 33; Lather Shave, 33; Medicated Face Conditioner, 36; Protein 21. See Protein 21; Protein 29. See Protein 29; Push Button Deodorant, 59; Shave Talc, 30; Skin Bracer, 36; Skin Bracer Pre-Electric Shave Lotion, 30; Sof' Stroke Regular Shave, 34; Speed Stick, 60
Menthol, 32, 35, 36, 149
Mermaid Ocean Sponge, 27
Methyl salicylate, 153
Mineral oil, 23, 27, 36, 68, 70–73, 98
Mini-peel, 77
Mink & Pearls: Cologne Concentrate spray, 55; Perfume, 51
Miss Dior: Eau de Cologne, 54; Perfume, 48
Mitchum: Cream Antiperspirant, 62; Non-Aerosol Antiperspirant, 61; Roll-On Antiperspirant, 62
Mitsouko: Cologne, 53; Perfume, 49

183

INDEX

Moisture level, 22
Moisturizers, 12–13, 16, 19, 22, 23, 66–74; aftersun, 165–166; brands, 67, 68, 70–73; common ingredients, 73–74
Monkey Brand, 87
Monsieur Houbigant, 46; Musk, 47
Mon Triomphe, 47
Moon Drops: Bronze Lustre, 163; Discovery Night Cream, 78
Mouthwash, 87–88
Multi-Scrub, 147
Musk Oil: Cologne Concentrate Spray, 55; for Men, 46; Perfume, 51
Myrurgia Perfumes. *See* Maja
My Sin: Eau liquid cologne, 54; Perfume, 50

Nail files, 175–176
Nail polishes, 108–109
Nail polish removers, 110–111
Nails, 107–114
Nail scissors and nippers, 175
Nair, 38
Narcisse Noir: Parfum de toilette, 53; Perfume, 49
"Natural" products, 3–4
Natural Sponge, 27
Natural Wonder: Keep Blushing, 100; Lipstick, 101; Oil-Free Pressed Powder, 99; Oil-Free Shear Makeup, 95; Shining Eyecrayon Pencil, 104; Shiny Shiny Lip Gloss, 102; Super Clean Up, 81–82
Nestlé: Balsam Plus Vitamin E Instant Hair Conditioner, 127; Noreen Color Rinse, 140; Protein Color Rinse, 140
Neutrogena: Acne Cleansing Soap, 147; Acne Drying Gel pH6, 145; Baby Soap, 17; basic formula, 12, 15; Dry Skin Soap, 17; Hand Cream, 75; Rainbath Dry Skin Bath Gel, 25
New Freshness, 64
New Organic Hair Remover Strips, 38
Night creams, 66–67, 78
Nina Ricci: colognes by, 55; perfumes by, 48, 49
Nippers, cosmetic, 175
Nivea, 43, 68; Creme Soap, 18
Norelco: Lady Norelco 20 L, 39; Ladyshave HP2108, 39; Rechargeable Tripleheader III Deluxe 45 CT, 39; Rechargeable Tripleheader VIP 50, 39; Speedshaver 11 20, 39; Tripleheader III 35 T, 39
Norell: Cologne, 51; Perfume, 48; Perfumed Milk Bath, 25; Soap, 21
Norwich Products, 153
Noxell. *See* Cover Girl; Noxzema
Noxzema: Brushless Shave Cream, 33; Cold Cream, 79; Liquid Skin Cream, 79; Medicated Lather

Noxzema *(cont'd)*
Shave Cream, 33; Regular Noxzema Skin Cream, 167; Skin Cream, 79
NP 27 Spray Powder, 153
Nuance: Cologne, 56; Perfume, 50
Nudit, 38; Cream Bleach for the Face, 141; Gentle Skin Lightener with Sunscreen, 81
Nuit de Noel: Parfum de toilette, 52; Perfume, 49
Nupercainal Pain Relief Lotion and Nupercainal Pain Relief Cream, 167
Nutraderm Dry Skin Lotion, 72
Nutraplus, 68

1–12, 45
Oatmeal and Bran Soap, 18
Ode, 48
Odorono Cream Deodorant Antiperspirant, 62
Ogilvie Conditioning Setting Lotion, 132
Oilatum, 17
Oil of bergamot, 3
Oil of Olay, 72
Oil of peppermint, 23
Oil of Peru, 3
Ointments, body, 75–76
Olay Vitalizing Night Cream, 78
Old Spice: After Shave, 37; After Shave Skin Conditioner, 36–37; Cologne for Men, 47; Deodorant, 59; Deodorant Powder, 60; Double Action Anti-Perspirant Deodorant, 61; Musk for Men After Shave Lotion, 37; Pre-Electric Shave Lotion, 30; Roll-On Antiperspirant Deodorant, 62; Shave Talc, 30; Shaving Mug Soap, 33; Stick Deodorant, 60
Orafix, 91
Oral-B, 89
"Organic" products, 3–4
Orlane: B 21 Creme Fluide for Body and Buste, 76; Creme B-21, 74; Flame Glo Makeup Moisture, 96; Lacta-Creme, 80; masks by, 170; "6 Carats" Nail Enamel, 109; Super Hydratante B 21, 78
Oster Mist Set, 177
Owen Labs: Ionax. *See* Ionax; Ionil. *See* Ionil; sunscreens by, 161

Paba, 60, 71, 160–165
Pabafilm Sunscreen Gel, 161
Pabagel Pure Paba Sunscreen Gel, 161
Pabanol, 161
Paco Rabanne, 45
Pacquin Hand Cream, 75; Medicated, 75
Padimate, 163, 164
Palmolive: Brushless Shave Cream, 33; Gold, 20–21; Lather Shave Cream, 33

Panasonic ES306 Durango, 39
Pancin, 157
Panoxyl-5 Gel and Panoxyl-10 Gel, 145
Pantene: Hair Spray De Pantene, 135; Heat Solution De Pantene, 128; Set De Pantene, 133; Shampoo for Fine or Thin Hair, 122
Para Labs, 169
Parfumerie, 21
Parfums Capucci, 45
Parfums Givenchy, Inc. *See* Givenchy; Givenchy III; Le De; L'Interdit
Parfums Gres. *See* Cabochard
Parfums Hermés: colognes by, 45, 52; perfume by, 48
Parfums Lagerfeld. *See* Chloe
Parfums Raphael. *See* Replique
Parfums Rochas: colognes by, 54; perfumes by, 49
Paris Presents, 47
Parke-Davis, 167
Patrick, 46
Peanut Oil, 71, 75
Pearl Drops Tooth Polish, 87
Pears Natural Transparent Soap, 17
Pencils: eye, 106; styptic, 35
Pennwalt Pharmacraft, 145
Pepsodent, 86–87
Perfumes, 41–51
Periodontitis, 84
Permanents, home, 140–141
Perma Tweez, 37, 176–177
Pernox Shampoo for Oily Hair, 122
Peroxide, 137
Persa-Gel 5% and Persa-Gel 10%, 145
Persistent light erupters, 20
Personna: Double II, 31; Double II Blades, 32; Lady, 31; 74 Tungsten Plus, 32
Perspiration, 20, 57–58, 149–151
Petrolatum (petroleum jelly), 19, 61, 68, 73–74, 75
Pfizer, Inc., 113
pH, 7, 11–12, 63–64, 119
Phisoac Cream, 145, 146
Phisoderm, 19
Phisohex, 19
Phototoxic reactions, 20, 33, 42, 43, 166
Physician's & Surgeon's Soap, 18
Pierre Cardin: after shave lotion, 37; Antiperspirant Deodorant, 62; cologne, 45
Pino Silvestre, 46
Plantar warts, 157
Plasti-Liner Temporary Denture Reliners, 91
Plough, Inc. *See* Coppertone; QT
Polident: denture adhesive, 90; denture cleaner, 90
Poli Grip, 91
Polly Bergen Company, 100
Polytar: Soap, 27; Shampoo, 124

184

INDEX

Pond's: Cold Cream, 79; Light Moisturizer, 72
Postinflammatory hyperpigmentation, 43–44
Pour un Homme, 46
Prell, 120
Preservatives, 7
Preshave preparations, 29–30
Presun 5% Paba Gel, 161
Prince Matchabelli: Cachet Moisturizing Hand and Body Lotion, 71; cologne by, 56; perfume by, 50
Princess Marcella Borghese: Clay Masque, 170; Clean Skin Simply Scrub, 23; Principessa Lipstick, 102
Pristeen Feminine Hygiene Deodorant Spray Powder, 63
Pro: Flair Style Hairbrush, 174; Styling Brush, 174
Procter and Gamble, 20, 124
Professional Cosmetics, 113
Propa pH, 147
Propylene glycol, 35, 36, 71–74
Protein, 121, 126
Protein 21: Conditioner, 127; Hairspray, 135; pH Balanced Shampoo, 122
Protein 29: Creme Hair Groom, 132; Dry Control Formula, 136; Hair Groom, 131, 136
Psoriasis, 27
Puig/Barcelona: colognes by, 45, 52, 54; perfumes by, 48, 49
Purcellin, 17, 72, 74
"Pure" products, 3–4
Purex, 144
Purpose Shampoo, 123
Py-Co-Pay: Natural Bristle, 89; regular model, 89; Softex, 89

QT: Foam, 164; Lotion, 164
Queen Helene Mint Julep Masque, 169
Quinsana: Deodorant Foot Powder, 150; Foot Deodorant Spray Powder Antiperspirant, 151; Plus Medicated Foot Powder, 152

Rain Tree Moisture with NPC, 72
Rapid Shave, 34; Cologne Scent, 34
Razor blades, 31–32
Razor bumps, 34–35
Razors: electric, 29, 39–40; nonelectric, 30–31
RD, 137
Redken Genuine Amino Pon Shampoo, 122
Reedco, Inc., 124
Remington: blow driers by, 178; Lady Remington LR70M, 39; LB30 Lektro Blade Shaver, 39; LBX Lektro Blade Shaver, 39; Princess CL50, 39
Replique: Eau de toilette, 56; Perfume, 50
Resorcinol, 145

Revlon: Aquamarine Conditioning Creme Rinse, 127; Body Silk Body Moisturizer, 71; Charles Revson. See Charles Revson; Charlie. See Charlie; Clean and Clear Deep Moisture Face Cleanser, 79; colognes by, 45, 46, 55, 56; Extra Life Top Coat, 113; Flex. See Flex; Frost Formula, 101; Hi & Dri Roll-On Antiperspirant, 62; Highlight White Vanishing Stick, 98; Milk Plus 6 Cleanser, 80; Milk Plus Six Shampoo & Conditioner, 122; Milk Plus 6 24-Hour Moisturizer, 72; Nail Tip Whitener, 114; Natural Herb Cleanser, 80; Natural Wonder Division. See Natural Wonder; Oxy-5 Acne Lotion, 144; Professional Setting Lotion, 132; Snow Silk Lightener, 137; Soap, 21; Super Sealer, 113; Super Skin Double Action Natural Cleanser for Oily Skin, 79–80; Toner for Normal to Dry Skin, 82; tweezers by, 175; Ultra Silk Hair Lightener, 137; Wonder Nail Nail Fortifier, 113
Rexall Redi-Shave Cream, 34
Rezamid Acne Lotion, 145, 146
R-gen Protein Hair Repair, 122
Rich Mer: Cocoa Butter Cream, 72; Original Vitamin-E-100 Vanishing Cream, 72
Right Guard: Anti-Perspirant, 60; Deodorant, 59; Deodorant Stick, 60; Double Protection Anti-Perspirant, 60; Double Protection Anti-Perspirant Roll-On, 62; Dry Talc Deodorant, 60; Powder Dry, 63; Pump Spray Anti-Perspirant, 61
Riker Labs, 147
Rise, 33; Baby Face, 33; Heavy, 33
Rive Gauche: Cologne, 56; Gentle Spray Deodorant, 59–60; Moisturizing Body Lotion, 76
Roger & Gallet: colognes by, 46, 56; perfume by, 50; soaps by, 21
Rose Milk Skin Care Cream, 72
Royal Copenhagen: after shave lotion, 37; cologne, 46
Rubifactant mask, 77, 170–171
RV Paba Lipstick, 161
RVP Wide-Spectrum Sunscreen, 163

Safe Dry Solid Antiperspirant, 62
Safeguard, 20
Safflower oil, 72
Salicylic acid, 36, 153, 156
Salicylic Acid and Sulfur Soap, 28, 146
Salicylic acid plaster, 153
Salicylic Acid Soap, 27
Sardo Bath Oil Concentrate, 25
Sastid Soap, 146

Satura Moisture Cream with Vitamin A, 72
Scalpmaster 100% Pure Boar Bristle, 174
Scandia: cheek blushers by, 100; Fluitone Makeup Foundations for Normal and Oily Skin, 97; Integra Eye Shadoliner, 105; Make-a-Tint Makeup Foundation, 97; mascaras by, 105; Retouch Cover-Up Cream, 98; Stimulus Natural Clay Masque, 170; Ultra Chexit, 62
Scannon Ltd., 46
Schering-Plough, 6
Schick: blow driers by, 178; Hot Lather Dispenser, Aerosol Refills for, 34; Injector, 30–31; Jewel by Lady Schick, 39; Lady Schick Quick Curls, 177; Lady Schick Shaving Wand, 39; Plus Platinum Blades, 32; Plus Platinum Teflon Coated Blades, 32; Staysharp SS11, 39; Superchromium Blades, 32; Superchromium With Teflon Coating, 32; Super II Blades, 32
Scholl. See Dr. Scholl's
Scissors, cosmetic, 175
Score: Micro-Emulsion Hair Groom, 131; Natural Hair Spray, 136
Scotchbrand Hairset Tape, 134
SD alcohol, 40, 75, 135, 136
Sea & Ski: Dark Tanning Oil, 163; Golden Tan, 163; Indoor/Outdoor Tanning Lotion, 164; Suntan Lotion, 162
Sea Breeze Antiseptic for the Skin, 167
Sebaceous skin oil, 12–13, 16, 69, 120, 142–143
Seba-Nil: Cleanser For Acne And Other Oily Skin Conditions, 81; Cleansing Mask, 169
Seborrhea, 27
Sebulex Medicated Shampoo, 124
Sebutone Therapeutic Tar Shampoo, 124
Selectra Cream Moisturizer, 68
Selenium, 123, 124
Selsun Blue, 124
Sensitization, 1–2, 6, 38
Sensodyne, 87
Sesame oil, 72
Setting lotions, 132–133
Shalimar: Cologne, 53; Perfume, 49
Shampoos, 12, 119–124
Shavex: Cordless Rechargeable XL400, 39; Lady Shavex 1700, 39
Shaving, 29–37
Shaving creams, 32–34
Shaving powder, 34–35
Shaving soaps, 33
Shepard's: Cream Lotion, 70; Moisturizing Soap, 18
Shine Offs Pure Linen Facial Blotters, 106

INDEX

Shulton, Inc. *See* Old Spice
Silicare Healing and Protective Lotion, 73
Silicone, 30, 34
Snug Denture Cushions, 91
Soaps, 11–28, 146–147
Sodium laureth sulfate, 121
Sodium lauryl sulfate, 64, 79
Sodium pyrithione, 132
Softique: Citrus Bouquet Bath Oil Beads, 25; Herbal Seas Bath Oil Beads, 25
Solarcaine Lotion and Solarcaine Spray, 167
Spa Genuine Loofah, 27
Speidel Textron, Inc., 47
Spray Neet Hair Remover, 38
Squibb, 6; 1600 Straight Handle Toothbrush, 89
Stearic acid, 70, 73
Stiefel Labs, 124, 145, 146
Styptic pencils, 35
Sudden Beauty Country Air Mask, 170
Sulfacet-R Lotion, 146
Sulfoxyl Lotion, 146
Sulfoxyl Lotion Regular and Sulfoxyl Lotion Strong, 145
Sulfur, 146, 147
Sulfur Soap, 146
Summer's Eve, 65
Sunbeam: blow driers by, 178; Shavemaster 5671, 39
Sunburn remedies, 166–167
Sun care products, 160–167
Sundare Sunscreen Creamy Lotion, 163
Sunscreens, 160–164
Suntans, 159–160, 164–165
Super Dry Sure, 61
Sure Long Lasting Antiperspirant Roll-On, 62
Surfactants, 86
Swank, Inc., 46, 47
Sweet almond oil, 72
Syntex Bath Oil, 25
Syosset Laboratories, 68

Tabac Blond: Parfum de toilette, 53; Perfume, 49
Talcum powder, 29; deodorant, 60; shaving, 30
Tallow, 17, 20
Tame Creme Rinse & Conditioner, 127
Tars, in dandruff shampoos, 123, 124
Teeth, 83–87
Teflon razor blade coatings, 32
Tegrin Medicated Shampoo, 124
Tek Professional, 89
Tender Touch Bath Oil, 25
Texas Pharmaceuticals, 145, 162
Thermodent, 87
Thicket, 130

Thick 'N Hair, 130
Thioglycolate, 34, 35, 38, 40
Tickle Roll-On Antiperspirant, 62
Tinactin, 152
Titanium dioxide, 98
Toenails, ingrown, 154
Toilet water, 41, 44, 51–56
Tolnaftate, 152
Tom's Natural Toothpaste, 87
Tone, 17, 19
Toni, 141
Toothbrushes, 89
Toothpaste, 85–87
Tooth powder, 85–87
Translucent makeup, 97
Trichloroacetic acid, 77
Triclocarban, 20–21
Triethanolamine, 36, 72, 74
Tropical Deluxe Formula Dark Tanning Oil, 162
Truc: Foaming Bath Gel, 25; Glycerine Soaps, 18
Truly Natural Face Color, 96
Tussy: Cream Deodorant Antiperspirant, 62; Roll-On Deodorant Antiperspirant, 62
Tweezers, cosmetic, 175
Twenty Carats: Eau de Parfum, 56; Perfume, 50

Ultima: Eau de toilette, 52; Liquid Skim Milk Soap, 21–22; Skim Milk Abrasive Cleanser, 22; Skim Milk Bath Oil, 25; Soap, 21
Ultra-Brite, 87
Ultrafine Nail-Strength Base Coat, 113
Undecylenic acid, 152
Urea, 68, 71, 74

Vagisec Douche Liquid Concentrate, 64
Vanseb Dandruff Shampoo with Protein, 124
Vaseline: Camphor Ice Skin Balm, 167; Hair Tonic and Scalp Conditioner, 131; Intensive Care Lotion, 73; Intensive Care Lotion Extra Strength for Problem Hands, 75; Pure Petroleum Jelly, 67, 74, 76, 77, 78, 98, 100, 101, 110, 111, 113
Vergo, 157
Ver-Var, 158
Vick Chemical Co. *See* Clearasil
Victor of Milano, 45
Vidal Sassoon: Non-Aerosol Hair Mist, 135; shampoos by, 122
Vistron-Pro, 174
Vitabath Gelée, 25
Vitalis: Clear Gel Greaseless Hair Groom, 130; Dry Texture for Men's Hair, 130; Dry 3 Hair Control, 136; Regular Hold, 135; With V 7, 131

Vol de Nuit: Cologne, 53; Perfume, 49

Warner-Lambert. *See* Listerex
Wart remedies, 155–158
Waxing preparations, 38
Wella: Balsam Conditioning Shampoo, 122; Balsam Instant Conditioner, 128; Flex. *See* Flex; Gentle Care Instant Hair Conditioner, 127; In-Depth Conditioning Treatment for Problem Hair With Provitamin B 5 and Protein, 128; Kolestral, 128
Wernet's Denture Adhesive Powder, 90
Westwood Pharmaceuticals: acne preparations by, 141, 146, 147; shampoos by, 122, 124; sunscreens by, 161
Wet and Set Treated Curl Papers, 134
Wheat germ oil, 72
Whiteners, nail-tip, 114
Whitehall Laboratories, 38, 170
Wibi Dry Skin Lotion, 73
Wildroot Creme Oil, 131
Wilkinson: Blades, 32; II Blades, 32; Bonded Blades, 32; Bonded System, 31; Swordmaster Chromium Blades, 32
Williams: Golden Yellow Lather Shaving Cream, 33; 'Lectric Shave, 30; 'Lectric Shave Tender Face Special Formula, 30; men's cologne by, 47; Mug Shaving Soap, 33
Winarick, A. R., Inc., 175, 176
Winthrop Labs, 145, 146
Witch hazel, 81, 82
Woodbury After Shave, 37
Wrinkle creams, 66–67, 76–77

Y: Eau de toilette, 52; Perfume, 48
Yardley: Clear Cover Slicker Nail Polish, 109; Deodorant for Men, 60; Old English Lavender Fragranced Soap, 21; Original After Shave, 37; Original Cologne, 47; Portrait Liquid Makeup, 96; Pot O Gloss, 102; Roll-on Antiperspirant Deodorant, 62
Yatagan, 45
Youth Hair, 137
Yves Saint Laurent: cologne by, 52; for Men, 45; perfume by, 48; shampoos by, 122

Zest, 20
Z-14, 45
Zincon Dandruff Shampoo, 124
Zinc oxide, 75, 98, 162
Zinc pyrithione, 123, 124, 132
Zip Depilatory Wax, 38
Zonite Liquid Douche Concentrate, 64